W9-BIU-751

FAMILY HEALTH:
FROM DATA TO POLICY

Edited by
GERRY E. HENDERSHOT, PH.D.
FELICIA B. LECLERE, PH.D.

Proceedings from a conference on
family data and family health policy
sponsored by the National Center for
Health Statistics, Public Health Service,
U.S. Dept. of Health and Human Services

Published by

National Council on Family Relations
Minneapolis, MN

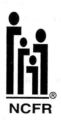

NCFR

ST. OLAF COLLEGE LIBRARIES

RA
418.5
.F3
F36
1993

The National Council on Family Relations was established in 1938 as a multi-disciplinary professional association to provide a forum for family researchers, educators, and practitioners to share in the development and dissemination of knowledge about families and family relationships, to establish professional standards, and to promote family policies that enhance their well-being. NCFR is privately supported through its members and sale of publications and educational programs. Beneficiaries of NCFR services include family professionals, policy makers and educators.

Library of Congress Cataloging-in-Publication Data

Hendershot, G. E., and LeClere, F.B.
ISBN-0-916174-37-9
Library of Congress Catalogue Card Number: 93-86892

Copyright © 1993 by the National Council on Family Relations.
All rights reserved. Printed in the United States of America. No part of this publication may be reproduced, stored in a retrieval system, or transmitted in any form or by any means, electronic, mechanical, photocopying, recording, or otherwise, without prior written permission of the publisher.

National Council on Family Relations
3989 Central Avenue NE, Suite 550
Minneapolis, MN 55421
612-781-9331
FAX 612-781-9348

30901029

Contents

Summary:

Foreword

During the past year, the Office of the Assistant Secretary for Planning and Evaluation (ASPE) in the Department of Health and Human Services, and the National Center for Health Statistics (NCHS) in the Centers for Disease Control and Prevention have undertaken several new activities to improve federal statistics on families. The activities were our response to the growing consensus in public policy debate that family issues are central to many of the nation's health and welfare problems, and our awareness that the federal statistical system was not well-prepared to respond to the data needs of that policy debate.

At ASPE, the Division of Family, Community, and Long-term Care Policy has done several things. First, it conducted an inventory of the family data systems in the federal government, and will soon publish a guide to those systems. The guide will enable researchers to find the family data that are available, and it will make clear what the gaps and shortcomings in our family data are. Second, the division has conducted systematic literature reviews of family studies in the major fields of health and welfare policy. Reports on those reviews will be published soon, and they will show that, disappointingly, the family has not been a focus of research in some policy areas where its importance would seem obvious, such as in education.

Third, the Division of Family and Community Policy has sponsored and organized an interagency Family Data Workgroup with members representing more than a dozen agencies in the Department of Health and Human Services, the first

such effort of its kind. The Workgroup meets monthly to exchange information on family statistics systems, and to coordinate and collaborate on initiatives in the field. Staff of NCHS have been active participants in the Workgroup.

At NCHS, family health statistics activities have been led by the Division of Health Interview Statistics, but staff of other data systems also have been involved. The Division is in the early stages of developing a survey on family and health issues to be fielded as part of the National Health Interview Survey (NHIS).

In preparation for that survey, a number of activities are underway. First, analyses using existing NHIS data are being published to meet as many data needs as possible. Second, through a series of Seminars on Family and Health, the family health data needs of the federal government are being assessed.

Third, a group of nationally eminent experts on family and health has been retained to provide advice on the kinds of questions and methods that can and should be included in a national survey. Finally, focus groups consisting of NCHS volunteers have been formed to help the NHIS staff understand the kinds of real world health experiences families are facing. While the NCHS activities are focused on the NHIS, they are benefiting other center data systems also.

As a result of these preliminary activities, we are convinced that the family has important effects on the health of its members in several ways: by creating the physical and psychological environment in which family members spend most of their time; by teaching and reinforcing behaviors that protect against or increase the risk of disease; and by providing home health care and access to professional health care. While we have good statistics on the environment, behavior, and care of individuals, our statistics on their effect in and through families are poor.

The activities of ASPE and NCHS are complimentary and mutually supportive. Recognizing their mutual interest, the two offices entered into an interagency agreement to co-sponsor and co-fund a Workshop on Family Data and Family Health Data. Subsequently, the Office of the Assistant Secretary for Health in the Department of Health and Human Services joined this effort as a co-sponsor, recognizing its particular needs for better family health statistics. The purposes of the Workshop were to increase the awareness of the need to improve federal statistics on families in general, and on family and health issues in particular, and to begin to form a consensus on what family and health statistics are needed. The in-tended audience was the federal agencies that need data for making health policy decisions, the federal agencies that fund research related to family health issues, and the research community that does (or should be doing) such research.

By choice and necessity, the Workshop was relatively small, with about 60 registered participants representing about 40 different government and private sector organizations. Because the Workshop began the day after a record breaking snowstorm, many participants had to make heroic efforts to attend. Those who made it were able to participate in a workshop that was, in the opinion of most of those present, unusually productive. The wide variety of backgrounds and experience among the participants, combined with their shared commitment to improving family data, created a synergy and excitement that we hope will be shared by the readers of these proceedings.

Gerry E. Hendershot
Felicia B. LeClere

MANNING FEINLEIB, M.D., PH.D.
Director, National Center for Health Statistics
Centers for Disease Control and Prevention

Introduction

This is an important time in the history of health care in the United States. We have achieved a national consensus that health care reform is needed, and the new administration has made such reform a central part of its plans. A task force is at work preparing a health care reform package that is scheduled for completion by May. Whatever its final form may be, we know the issues it will address: access to medical care, containment of medical care costs, and health promotion and disease prevention.

The Centers for Disease Control and Prevention are playing an important role in planning for these changes. As part of CDC,

> "The mission of the National Center for Health Statistics is to provide statistical information that will guide actions and policies to improve the health of the American people. As the Nation's principal health statistics agency, NCHS leads the way with accurate, relevant, and timely data."

We do so by operating an integrated set of more than a dozen data systems, including the Mortality Statistics system, the National Health and Nutrition Examination Survey, the National Health Interview Survey, and the National Health Care Survey.

To fulfill our mission to provide relevant and timely data, NCHS must anticipate and prepare for future data needs. In that spirit, members of our staff began more than two years ago to assess the need for family-related health statistics. It seemed to us that many of the emerging issues of access, cost, and prevention were also family issues, and our data systems needed to reflect this emerging trend.

We found support for our efforts elsewhere in CDC and the Department of Health and Human Services. For instance, CDC has established a Family, Infant, and Child Health Workgroup to share information and coordinate research and program activities. The Office of the Assistant Secretary for Planning and Evaluation, ASPE, in the Department of Health and Human Services, established an interagency Family Data Workgroup to assess data needs. And now ASPE and the Office of the Assistant Secretary for Health have joined NCHS in sponsoring this workshop.

What do we expect to accomplish in this workshop? What we expect to do here is to identify the major data needs for emerging family-related health policy issues. What health policy issues have a specific and significant family aspect? What health statistics are needed to inform policy discussion about those issues? And finally, what practical next steps can we recommend to see that those family-related health data are available when they are needed?

You were invited to this conference because we believe that you can help us to answer those questions. You represent government statistical agencies, government policy offices, private sector family agencies, and the academic research community. You are here because you share an interest in family-related public health issues, and a conviction that good data are essential to making and implementing sound public health policy.

So that we may focus your time and talents on the central purposes of this workshop, let me briefly point out what this workshop is not about. This is not a workshop on the substance of family-related health policy; debate on alternative policies will be carried out in other forums. Neither do we expect to solve some of the knotty methodological problems in family health statistics, such as defining and measuring family structure; we are addressing those problems in other projects. Finally, we do not expect to develop a detailed agenda for scientific research on family-related health issues; the National Institute for Child Health and Human Development is taking the lead in that effort.

During this workshop experts from several disciplines will discuss the interactions between family and health. Let me begin that discussion by suggesting several ways that the family affects the health of its members. A successfully functioning family contributes to the good health of its members by creating a healthy physical and psychological *environment* for its members; by teaching and reinforcing healthy *behaviors* by its members; and by providing home care or access to medical *care* for its members.

A particularly alarming example of the family's potential to create an unhealthy *physical environment* for its members is cigarette smoking. Medical research has established that exposure to secondary smoke—passive smoking—increases the risks of respiratory and other diseases. Yet data from our National Health Interview Survey show that one-half of preschool aged children have been exposed to secondary smoke in the family. Of the exposed children, most were exposed to the smoking of their mother during her pregnancy *and* to the smoking of adults in the family after their birth.

In addition to affecting the health of the environment in which its members live, the family also teaches and reinforces health-related *behaviors* by its individual members. Sometimes children learn the unhealthy behavior exemplified by older family members. For instance, an NCHS survey of adolescent tobacco use found that adolescents were 30 percent more likely to initiate cigarette smoking if their parents smoked than if their parents did not smoke. The influence of older siblings in the family was even stronger: adolescents were twice as likely to initiate smoking if they had an older sibling who smoked than if they did not.

In the debate about our national health care system, the important role of the family as a provider of *home care* in that system is too often overlooked. For instance, family members comprise the majority of care givers for our dependent elderly citizens: the National Health Interview Survey shows that three-fourths (75 percent) of dependent persons 70 years of age and older receive home care from family members.

The role of the family in health is especially important at this time in our history, because trends in family formation and dissolution are creating new diversity in our family types. Modern families are of many different structural types: the "traditional" type with once-married parents and their biological children; the "melded" family with previously married parents and biological and step-children; the never-married, single parent family; the single parent formerly married family; and many more.

The effects of these changes in family types on the health of family members are not well understood, but some of the evidence is disturbing. For instance, in a study based on the National Health Interview Survey, it was found that the health of children was least vulnerable if they were living in a "traditional" family with both biological parents. Their health was most vulnerable if they were living with their never-married mother and no father.

In this same study, the findings for childhood injuries were especially ominous. As you know, among children and adolescents, injury is the leading cause of chronic impairment and mortality. The incidence of injury was lowest among children in "traditional" families—13 percent were injured in the year before interview. The incidence of injury was 19 percent higher among children in mother-stepfather families, and 31 percent higher among children of formerly married mothers with no father present.

What explains such differences in health status and behavior among family types? Right now, we really don't know, because our health data systems have tended to focus on the individual, not the family. Consequently, we know relatively little about the details of family social structures and processes, and we are not in a good position to explain differences in their health outcomes.

We think we can improve our data on family-related health issues, and I have indicated some of the efforts we already are making in that direction. To help us do that, I ask again that during these two days together you help us to identify the major data needs for emerging family-related health policy issues. What health policy issues have a specific and significant family aspect? What health statistics are needed to inform policy discussion about those issues? And finally, what practical next steps can we recommend to see that those family-related health data are available when they are needed?

FRANCES GOLDSCHEIDER, PH.D.
Professor of Sociology
Brown University

The Changing American Family and Public Health Policy: Gender and Intergenerational Relationships in the Context of Demographic Change

This paper was written while in residence as a Research Associate at RAND, Santa Monica, California.

I. INTRODUCTION

We all know that the American family has been changing. It has always been changing, so it is not change, itself, that is new. What I can try to contribute is to frame recent trends within a context of changing intergenerational and male-female relationships, to elucidate some of the causes behind the patterns of change that have emerged, and cast the whole within a health policy context. In doing so, I will consider something that I think is genuinely new, highlighting the often overlooked role of the growth in non-family living in these changes.

To do so, I will have to ground my remarks in a brief excursion into the major processes of demographic change and link them to recent social and family history, since it is my view that responses to these trends underlay many of the "ills" of the family most of us are concerned about. The demographic change that is central is the revolution in "joint survivorship," which is

the engine that has been transforming adult and family-related roles for over a century. But our recent family history is rooted in the myths of the 1950s, when massive resistance to the consequences of the demographic changes led to an extreme of gender role segregation which did harm while it was in place, and, in crashing around us, is doing more harm and creating new myths, as I will try to document. The challenge I will pose to family policy makers is to highlight the costs these myths create and to work with the underlying processes of change to hasten a sustainable and sustaining resolution.

II. JOINT SURVIVORSHIP

First let us think about the rise of joint survivorship, which simply means the increased duration of family relationships that has become possible because of the decline in mortality. We now take for granted the revolution in health and survival that has nearly doubled life expectancy in this century. But it is only in our immediate lifetimes that the impact has accumulated of the enormous lengthening of family relationships, both relationships between those of the same generation and those of different generations. And as a longer life has led to a qualitative restructuring of our

4

individual lives, with time for extended education, for a lengthy retirement, for developing a second career or a second family, so, too, does the lengthening of our relationships change them not just in duration, but in kind. Transformations are in progress in parent-child relationships and male-female relationships. In the process, father-children relationships are at risk, but we will build up to that in due time.

A. Joint Survivorship and Parent-Child Relationships

Let me give a quick example about parent-children relationships. On average, women can now expect their mothers to live 55 years after their own birth (Mencken, 1985). This means that nearly two-thirds of the time parents and children live together on this earth are spent when both are adults. This has really upset transitions for family businesses—farm and non-farm—as well as for royal governments where children are not supposed to assume an adult level of control until their parents' death or frailty. Think—a "child" may have to wait to age 50 or 60 or beyond to assume hereditary responsibilities.

Even when there is no business or farm to take into account, the same dynamics apply. The kind of parent-child relationship that makes sense while children are young is not comfortable or supportive when it is between two mature adults. Hence, the extension of joint survivorship requires a transition in the structure of parent-child relationships to retain the benefits of this historic and powerful tie.

As yet, few parents who now have grown children had models for such a transition in their relationships with their own parents. Some women are beginning to reach for a more "sisterly" relationship with their daughters, and somewhat fewer men are learning to become "partners" with their sons, but we still have a considerable way to go before this transition becomes normal and comfortable, in part because few define it as anything other than a personal issue. Yet it is a genuine social problem, as well, since as parents and as adults with parents, most of us are struggling with this revolution in one way or another, sometimes exercising too little authority over our small children and sometimes feeling rebellious when our aging parents try to exercise too much authority. All change is difficult, but in this case, I doubt that we will want to reverse course. What

would be better is to learn as a society how to negotiate this transition.

B. Male-Female Relationships and the Loss of Fatherhood

In contrast, the male-female relationship, which is between two adults, has become fraught with transitions of a nearly gymnastic quality as a result of the extension of joint survivorship. The same calculations that allow us to see that the parent-child relationship will normally survive long into the child's adult years demonstrate that the connection between marital and parental roles must also loosen. Men and women who marry in their twenties or early thirties and have an average of two children can expect their marital relationship to survive until long after the children are grown and are actively involved in their own parental and even grandparental roles. The "empty nest" stage, which was once rarely achieved, is now the rule in marriages that survive divorce (Glick & Parke, 1965).

Thus parenthood can no longer be the major focus of adults' family lives, but the unfolding of this reality led to some amazing contortions. As demographic changes made the lives of men and women increasingly similar, 20th century Western societies reacted against this trend with a broad range of responses. In the United States, the response that was the most prominent was to maximize the remaining differentiation in men's and women's roles by assigning nearly all parenting responsibilities to women.

Whereas in the 17th and 18th centuries, men were primarily responsible for the practical and moral education of their children, this began to erode in the 19th century as the movement of men out of the home to more distant work sites gave women the leverage and the incentive to take over, leaving men with little more than the responsibility to provide and perhaps to spank. Much as obstetricians in the face of a shrinking market for baby delivering were able to drive out midwives by professionalizing (Kobrin, 1966), many women actively resisted the decline in their parenting roles by monopolizing parenthood and pursuing domesticity. This insured that the opportunities to earn cash in the emerging urban-industrial economy were disproportionately developed to replace men's subsistence contributions and not women's. It also meant that women were participating in a process that I feel has reconfigured the American family in such a way that a fault

6

line runs through it, with men on one side and women and children on the other. And it is currently a fault of San Andreas potential.

Women's increased specialization in parenting also created a life course trajectory for them that had several distinct "segments" and hence a marriage trajectory for men and women together marked by built-in radical transformations. If we were to describe the "ideal" life course stages of a marriage of the 1950s, they would include: (1) both partners childless but most wives no longer employed, a transition for women from full-time student or worker; (2) parenthood, with women redefining themselves as childraisers and drastically increased male financial responsibility; (3) the empty nest, as women "retired" from daily parenthood, and to a less productive role, if they hadn't returned to work; and finally (4) the husband's retirement. But throughout, women would have the additional responsibility of making the home for them all. If one re-negotiation is difficult for parent-child relationships, think what four do to the quality and strength of the marital tie. But we didn't recognize this fraying over the growing fault line, because with the decline in the

production value of women's work in the home, men's incomes had become increasingly necessary to them. So women were expected to be social gymnasts in the ideal marriage of the 1950s.

But as we know, this delicate situation was not destined to last, since women's problem of having no income was about to end. Female labor force participation began to increase rapidly, both around their shrinking childrearing responsibilities and in combination with them, as the logic of raises, benefits, pension vesting, and so forth made women increasingly aware of the costs to them of a segmented work strategy. This trend begins to make men's and women's lives more similar again, in recognition of the new demographic reality. Figure 1 shows data on labor force participation rates for currently married women, which begins in 1947 with very low rates overall and particularly for those with children < 6.

The data point for those without children < 18 would be higher if we could have excluded women 65+.

Then you see the dramatic increase for married women with children of all ages, reaching nearly 70% for those with school age children, al-

FIGURE 1. LABOR FORCE PARTICIPATION RATES FOR CURRENTLY MARRIED WOMEN AGED 16+, WITH AND WITHOUT CHILDREN UNDER AGE 18: 1948–1991.

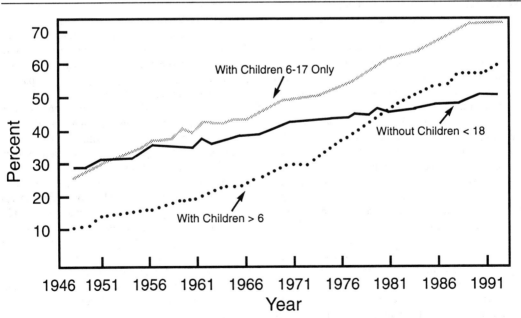

Source: Bureau of Labor Statistics 1980, 1989;
U.S. Bureau of the Census, 1991a, 1992e.

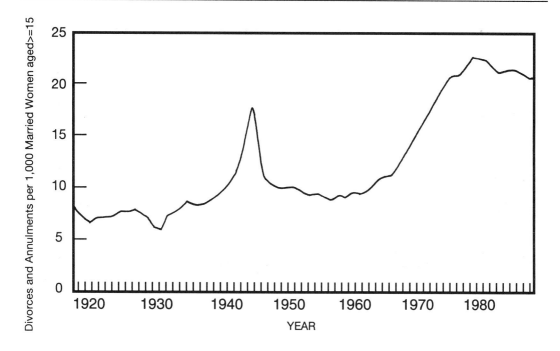

FIGURE 2. TREND IN DIVORCE: 1920–1988

Source: National Center for Health Statistics, 1991a.
          1988 data were obtained from NCHS over the Phone

though the level for those with pre-school-age children remains substantially lower, likely in response to the lack of appropriate child care for them. These trends seem to be moving upward, inexorably, like the increase in joint survivorship, and I know of no society around the world that has seen this trend reverse.

As a result, the disruption in male-female relationships, which began with the response to the extension of joint survival that created violent swings in marital roles, has allowed the exit of men from family roles. With manhood increasingly defined only in terms of accomplishments outside the family and with the loss of most of men's active parenting role, strains in marriage translate quickly to disaster for fatherhood. Figure 2 shows the trend in divorce from 1920 to 1988.

Divorce is normally seen only as rupturing the male-female relationship, but we now know it is responsible for a great loss in father-child relationships, based on studies of contact between non-coresident fathers and their children (Furstenberg & Nord, 1985).

The role of fathers in the family is not only declining because of divorce, when the children at least have some hope to maintain an existing relationship, but also via the growth of parenthood to unmarried women. Figure 3 shows that their birth rates have increased from less than one-seventh those of married women to nearly half their level.

It seems to me that the one point missing in the "Murphy Brown" debate was: why is it so realistic for Murphy, and for so many nonfictional women, to give up on finding a man to share parental responsibilities with? Because there are too few men who see active parenting as desirable, and who want to enter into an egalitarian relationship in order to do so. A century of transformation of the male role brought them to that point, and too many men are still locked in that 1950s definition. Families may need fathers, but men don't need to father. At least, they don't think they do.

III. THE FAMILY CONSEQUENCES OF FAMILY CHANGE

The separation of men from the mother-child unit as a result of the increase in divorce and out-of-wedlock parenthood has had drastic

8

FIGURE 3. BIRTH RATES FOR WOMEN, BY MARITAL STATUS: 1940–1989

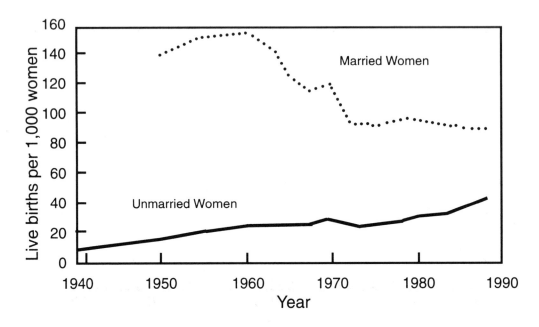

Source: National Center for Health Statistics, 1990, 1991b.
Note: Data refer to women aged 15-44.The birth rate for unmarried women is live births per 1,000 unmarried women. The birth rate for married women is live births per 1,000 married women. Data are estimated for years 1940-1979. Data are reported/inferred for years 1980-1989. Data are unavailable for married women before 1950.

financial consequences for children. Despite the increase in female labor force participation, women have not reached parity with men in the number of years they have worked by a given age, or the number of hours per week or weeks per year they work. And far more problematically, the jobs they do hold pay far less than those held by men.

Figure 4, which presents median family incomes in 1991 by family type, shows the results of these inequalities for children.

It is much better, financially, for children to live in a two-parent household, since married-couple families with children under 18 have the highest median incomes in the figure. But more than 25% of families with children (data not presented) have only one parent. A small group of these (about one-sixth) live with fathers only, in households with 56% as much income as two-parent families. But the vast majority of children living in single-parent families are living with their mothers, with family incomes only 30% as great as children living with two parents.

These averages are really only a snapshot of the relationship between income and family struc-

ture, which many thought was a misleading view. For a long time, scholars following the trend in divorce were reassured that the periods of living with a single parent were quite brief, a "time of transition" followed by nearly commensurate increases in remarriage, which seemed to "heal" the fracture. Calculations based on current income (Hoffman & Duncan, 1988) were reassuring, since clearly substantial proportions of the women and children who fell into poverty were removed by marriage.

If the definition of the co-resident father role has become attenuated, as I have argued here, the evidence suggests that the non-coresident father role is even more attenuated, and the role of the stepfather is virtually nonexistent, with matters to be negotiated among the respective parties as private solutions. These negotiations do not appear to lead to a strong stepfather-stepchild relationship when the children grow up (Cooney & Uhlenberg, 1990). More critically, we know that remarriage does not make up many of the financial losses children of divorce experience, since they are losers in terms of the financing of college education (Goldscheider & Goldscheider, 1991) and

FIGURE 4. 1991 MEDIAN INCOMES OF HOUSEHOLD, BY TYPE AND PRESENCE OF RELATED CHILDREN UNDER AGE 18

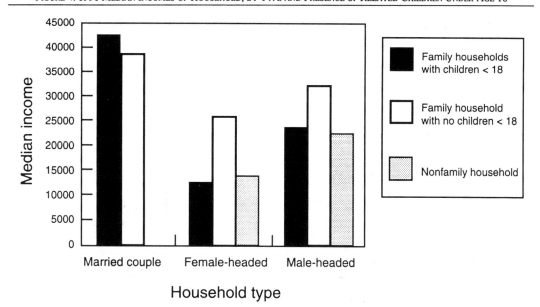

Household type

eventual status attainment (Biblarz & Raftery, 1993). Children may share in the life style their stepfather's income allows, but evidently they are not invested in the way they might have been from a father's income. And we know children experience major social and emotional strains from divorce and remarriage that are reflected in a wide range of problematic symptoms which we will discuss later in this workshop. So we need to know much more about what stepparents contribute—and how to help them build on their access to children to parent effectively.

IV. THE FLIGHT FROM THE FAMILY

An important lesson I have tried to convey in this review is that it is important, in studying family change, to note not only how families are changing, but also to note who isn't there, as a result, and what this might mean. So I have highlighted the increasing marginality of men in the family, particularly as fathers, with consequences for the health of women and children that we will focus on in the sessions to come because men and male incomes are not there. But I also think we should focus on what the costs might be for men as a result of the attenuation of their family roles. This requires us to consider a phenomenon rarely considered in studies of family change, which is that 25% of American households now contain only one person. This is a rapidly growing group of

people who "aren't there" because they are living outside family relationships altogether.

This trend began with the elderly. Figure 5 shows the growth in non-family living among women aged 60 and over between 1950 and 1980, which would look even more dramatic if we focused on the unmarried.

The trend toward non-family living has always seemed benign in the context of studying changes in the living arrangements of the elderly, since when we focus on the older generation, the decline in intergenerational coresidence allows us to continue to deny, under the rubric of "independence and dignity for life," that the life course includes a segment of increasing dependence and death. And when we focus on the younger generation, and see them living outside family relationships for a decade or more between high school and marriage, we also try to see this change as positive, since it allows us to avoid restructuring our adult parent-child relationships and confront our fears of domination. The maintenance of these two flights-from-reality unfortunately also allows us all to continue to deny that close family relationships are valuable, and that living alone is inevitably more expensive, often lonely, and occasionally dangerous.

Figure 6 shows how the growth in non-family living has been spreading to other parts of the life course, among adults aged 18 to 24 between 1950 and 1980 (which would also be much more dramatic if we removed the married).

FIGURE 5. LIVING ARRANGEMENTS OF WOMEN AGED 60 AND OLDER IN 1950 AND 1980

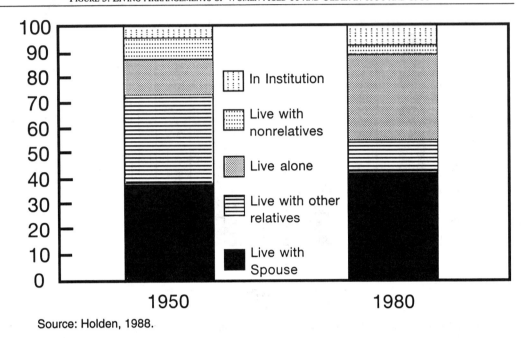

Source: Holden, 1988.

FIGURE 6. LIVING ARRANGEMENTS OF YOUNG ADULTS AGED 18–24 IN 1950 AND 1980

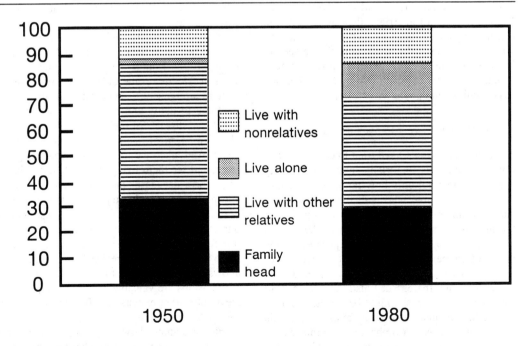

Because it is new and unstudied, non-family living among young people is also mysterious, with public confusion over recent trends and theoretical confusion about what it means for young adulthood and for the institution of the family. The recurring hysteria in the press about finding any unmarried adults living with their parents seems to suggest that non-family autonomy is increasingly required—that much of the press's readership feels that to live with parents after reaching some "adult" age, such as 18 or 21, is a sign of dangerous immaturity (e.g., Cowan, 1989; Gross, 1991) even though few would want most young adults to marry by these young ages.

Further, such press reports typically argue that the phenomenon of young adults remaining "in the nest" is increasing, when in fact, the likelihood that young unmarried adults would be living with their parents has declined and the proportion living alone has increased. What people are in fact noticing is the decline in the proportion forming new families, since the boom in family headship peaked in 1960, when large proportions of young adults were drawn into an independent residence via marriage, and then declined sharply, with some of the increase in non-marriage increasing the proportion of the total living in the parental home. But the proportion of the unmarried living away from the parental home has continued to increase.

Surprisingly little research has been done to show what the consequences might be of this increase in non-family living among young adults, I feel, because powerful American values about independence make the growth in non-family living among young adults also seem highly desirable. The lack of good research on this question is particularly critical, since young people have many years for any consequences to have their effect. There is evidence that living outside a family setting in young adulthood delays marriage and alters young people's attitudes toward several dimensions of traditional family roles (Goldscheider & Waite, 1991).

My guess is that there are often other costs of non-family living to young people's well-being, costs that parallel those of divorce. There is a direct link, since a wide range of recent evidence has documented that leaving home is earliest and non-family living highest among the children of divorce and remarriage (White & Booth, 1985; Mitchell et al., 1989; Aquilino, 1990; Goldscheider & Goldscheider, 1989; forthcoming). Those young adults leaving home experience a dramatic drop in household income when they leave their parental home, even after taking into account the lower need for income in their households (Hill, 1977). And they have less access to health insurance than any other group. It is also quite likely that they are spending on their rent earnings that could have been spent to further their educations and provide savings for an eventual home and family.

The health costs of non-family living at any age might be substantial, as well. Most evidence suggests that living with family is healthier, both mentally and physically. While many of those living outside a family setting may be able to construct a supportive network of social ties, many do not, risking loneliness, depression, and illness (Kobrin & Hendershot, 1977; Kisker & Goldman, 1987; Riessman & Gerstel, 1985).

V. CONCLUSION: THE GAINS TO RESTRUCTURING THE FAMILY

So what's a policy maker to do? What should be changed that can be changed? In any assessment of the appropriate responses of public policy to change in the private arena, the key question that must be asked is: what are the areas where policy can make a difference, and where does it have no impact, or even make things worse? We all know stories about commuter super highways constructed at great expense to reduce traffic congestion that rapidly became big parking lots, like the Beltway, as more people gave up on deteriorating public transportation systems. But we also know of policies that "work" as they were designed to, in which small financial investments reap large economic and social returns, like Head Start and WIC. I have tried to focus on the nature of the changes underway, so that we could all see which are largely irreversible and must be worked with, meliorating the costs of change as best we can; and which might not be sustainable, and should not be reinforced. I think that non-family is like the all purpose private car. It feels too independently wonderful to challenge, even when we see what it does to health, community, and the quality of life. And I think there is a lot we could do to reduce its incidence if we tried.

I think major gains in well-being could be made if we were able to make progress on both the gender and intergenerational fronts:

1. Integrate men back into the lives of their families. In a telling piece of research, Morgan et al. (1988) showed that divorce

rates in families with boy children were considerably lower than in those with only girl children. And despite the fact that they also showed that men are more involved with their children (male and female) when they had boys, no one has gotten past the shiver ("How sexist men are") to see and test the broader point: that men who are more involved in the lives of their children—sons and daughters—have more to lose from divorce, hence have more stake in negotiating marital differences successfully (for example, over housework), and therefore are more likely to have happier and more stable marriages. Thus the "family carrot" for men is a richer and more supportive family life. Policies that encourage men to actively father during their marriages, when it is much easier, will have the benefit of reducing the need to chase after absent fathers later. Think of it as preventive family health care.

And there is also a stick: we need more and better research to dramatize the established point that even more than women, men who live alone are at physical and mental health risk. Men feel that the homes their parents or wives provide for them include little that they could not easily replace. Homemaking skills are not highly valued, particularly by men, so they have little fear of living alone, and they have high expectations for remarriage, since we have managed not to inform them of the rapid decline in the male remarriage rate. They have been misled.

2. I also think that there are ways to re-integrate the generations safely back into each others' lives, so that the elderly can gain the benefits of close relationships with their grown children, and young people do not have to leave home in order to feel like an adult. Policies that reinforce family living arrangements will accelerate these negotiations, as well.

The most dangerous policy is to ignore the growth in non-family living. We are letting its superficial attractiveness as a source of "independence" blind us to its power to derail family change. It has become a diversion that allows us all to postpone indefinitely the renegotiations needed in inter-generational and male-female relationships that have become so necessary due to prolongation of joint survivorship. If we continue to ignore it, we risk losing the benefits to health and well-being of many of our closest and most supportive family relationships.

REFERENCES

Aquilino, W. (1990). The likelihood of parent-child coresidence: Effects of family structure and parental characteristics. *Journal of Marriage and the Family, 52*, 405-419.

Biblarz, T., & Raftery, A. (1993). The effects of family disruption on social mobility. *American Sociological Review, 58*, 97-109.

Cooney, T., & Uhlenberg, P. (1990). The role of divorce in men's relations with their adult children after mid-life. *Journal of Marriage and the Family, 52*, 677-688.

Cowan, A. L. (1989, March 12). Parenthood II: The nest won't stay empty. *The New York Times*, pp. 1, 30.

Furstenberg, F., & Nord, C. (1985). Parenting apart: Patterns of childrearing after marital disruption. *Journal of Marriage and the Family, 47*, 893-904.

Glick, P., & Parke, R. (1965). New approaches in studying the life cycle of the family, *Demography, 2*, 187-202.

Goldscheider, F., & Goldscheider, C. (1989). Family structure and conflict: Nest-leaving expectations of young adults and their parents. *Journal of Marriage and the Family, 51*, 87-97.

Goldscheider, F., & Goldscheider, C. (1991). The intergenerational flow of income: Family structure and the status of black Americans. *Journal of Marriage and the Family, 53*, 499-508.

Goldscheider, F., & Goldscheider, C. (forthcoming). *Leaving home before marriage*. University of Wisconsin Press.

Goldscheider, F., & Waite, L. (1991). *New families, no families? The transformation of the American home.* University of California Press.

Gross, J. (1991, June 16). More young single men hang onto apron strings: Recession and pampering keep sons at home. *The New York Times*, pp. 1, 18.

Hill, M. (1977). Sons and daughters. In G. Morgan & J. Morgan (Ed.), *Five Thousand American Families—Patterns of Economic Progress*, (Vol VI, pp. 117-146). University of Michigan, Institute for Social Research.

Hoffman, S., & Duncan, G. (1988). What are the economic consequences of divorce? *Demography, 25*, 641-645.

Kisker, E., & Goldman, N. (1987). Perils of single life and benefits of marriage. *Social Biology, 34*, 135-140.

Kobrin, F. E. (1976). The primary individual and the family: Changes in living arrangements since 1940. *Journal of Marriage and the Family, 38*, 233-239.

Kobrin, F. (1966). The American midwife controversy: A crisis of professionalization. Bulletin of the History of Medicine 40: 350-363. (REPRINTED IN: J. Leavitt and R. Numbers, eds., *Sickness and Health in America*. University of Wisconsin Press, 2nd ed., 1985.)

Kobrin, F., & Hendershot, G. (1977). Do family ties reduce mortality? Evidence from the United States, 1966-1968. *Journal of Marriage and the Family, 39*, 737-745.

Mencken, J. (1985). Age and fertility: How late can you wait? *Demography, 22*, 469-483.

Mitchell, B., Wister, A., & Burch, T. (1989). The family environment and leaving the parental home. *Journal of Marriage and the Family, 61*, 605-613.

Morgan, S. P., Lye, D., & Condran, G. A. (1988). Sons, daughters, and the risk of marital disruption. *American Journal of Sociology, 94*, 110-129.

Riessman, C., & Gerstel, N. (1985). Marital dissolution and health: Do males or females have greater risk? *Social Science and Medicine, 20*, 624-630.

White, L., & Booth, A. (1985). The quality and stability of remarriages: The role of stepchildren. *American Sociological Review, 50*, 689-698.

KARL ZINSMEISTER, PH.D.
Adjunct Scholar
American Enterprise Institute for Public Policy Research

Response to the Keynote Address by

Frances Goldscheider

I am pleased to be able to second the warning Professor Goldscheider serves up in her conclusion. It is true, as she says, that any time large numbers of citizens are living and growing up outside family settings, serious personal and societal problems will result. We have mounds of evidence showing that individuals lacking family moorings are likelier to become enmeshed in violence, substance abuse and poverty. They are more likely to experience mental illness, suicide and accidental injury. Dr. Goldscheider is certainly correct that we have no alternative but to renew and reinvigorate families — because there are no reliable substitutes on a mass scale for the emotional, economic, and psychological "services" that families render us. We simply cannot succeed as a society if most citizens choose to live outside these natural micro-communities. The irreplaceability of families is especially clear when you adopt the viewpoint of children. Some of the issues Professor Goldscheider raises — for instance her questions about the appropriate relationship between men and women within families — are in my opinion not really policy issues, but rather are items for individual couples to work out privately. The effect of family conditions on children, however, is clearly a legitimate concern of public policy. So in my remarks this afternoon I'll mostly address families from a child's-eye view. And I would like to begin by pointing out that from children's vantage, it is important not only

that families stay in favor, but that particular kinds of families stay in favor. The stark fact is that many of the so-called "new forms of family" that have evolved over the last generation have produced sharply negative effects on personal well-being, particularly child well-being.

To take just one example, we've recently learned that step-families are relatively poor substitutes for natural intact families. We have data showing that children growing up in step-families are far, far likelier to be abused, to drop out of school, to initiate early intercourse, to experiment with drugs and alcohol, to get in trouble with the law, and to end up with emotional and academic problems. Strikingly, children from step-families have a behavioral profile much more like that of single-parent children than like children from natural two-parent families. Indeed they even carry some extra disadvantages above and beyond those borne by single-parent children. Step-families may look benign when viewed as economic units. But their record shows that they provide no solution to the critical psychic problems that result from family breakdown.

So not only do families matter, specific types of families matter. In particular, there does not seem to be any easy substitute for the natural intact family. Given that four out of ten American children are living apart from at least one of their natural parents as we speak, this is a worrisome fact. Now — mindful of the fact that the over-arching purpose of this conference is to improve data collection, I want to zero in a little bit on the question of what it is we ought to be measuring when we approach families as analysts these days. I must tell you, there is something very liberating for me about knowing that everyone else in this room is as fascinated with social statistics as I am. I have been a little inhibited about confessing my interest in demographic data ever since the day a couple years ago when I told a long-lost attorney friend about the kind of work I did and he answered that he found that interesting, because he had heard social demographics was a field for people who liked numbers but didn't have enough personality to become accountants. This afternoon I guess we demographic bugs can let it all hang out. Which is good — because, as you all know, the way investigators measure and diagnose is going to have a lot to do with how they prescribe a little further down the road.

As for the particular case I want to argue this afternoon — if I had to reduce it to a bumper sticker it would come out something like this: If we want to get a better handle on how families and particularly children are now faring, we are going to have to shift our focus away from measurements of physical and material status, and look more closely instead at behavioral issues.

One reason I advocate such a shift is that many of the old battles have essentially been won. There is, for instance, practically no family hunger problem left in this country. We have good studies showing that the poor now take in virtually identical levels of protein, vitamins, and calories as high income Americans. Children living in poverty today are one inch taller and 10 pounds heavier than same-age children from the general population of the late 1950s. The main nutrition-related problem in America today is not under-feeding but rather obesity. In those few places where authentic nutritional problems linger — as among some homeless persons — they are linked to specialized mental health or drug addiction problems. There is no general hunger problem pressing down on American families today, and we ought to stop pretending otherwise.

There are lots of other more-or-less slain dragons which should now be dragged off center stage and over to the margins of national policy. Analysts worrying about the schoolability of American children used to look at things like the educational history of parents, and the number of other siblings an average child had to share his home with. On these traditional fronts, children are,

once again, far better off today as shown in Figures 1 & 2.

Likewise, amidst the concerns today about teen childbearing — children having children, as the slogan goes — the fact that the teenage birthrate is currently 35 percent lower than it was in 1960 gets overlooked as shown in Figure 3.

We no longer have a general problem with teen births in this country. What we have is a problem with illegitimate teen births (see Figure 4).

This is one of the behavioral issues I suggest we need to start looking at more specifically. The older, broader, material problems are no longer very relevant, so analysts and policy makers need to sharpen their focus. (In this regard it is interesting to note that the children of high income unmarried mothers have more health problems than the children of low income married mothers.)

Another aspect of family policy where far too much lumping and generalizing takes place is infant mortality. Figure 5 shows the U.S. infant mortality rate going back to 1940.

As you can see, there is not even a hiccup in this long line of improvement. We don't have an infant mortality crisis in this country.

What we do have is a significant but relatively narrow sector where behavioral and lifestyle choices — mostly drug addiction and smoking in underclass neighborhoods — are having seriously negative effects on pre-born children and neonates. The way to see that is not by tracing infant mortality rates but by looking at low birth weight rates. Figure 6 shows the changes since 1950.

In similar ways, I would argue that our national statistics on family poverty are not especially useful today. You can find out more interesting things about the material condition of households by using consumer expenditure data for the lowest quintile (which, by the way, shows low income Americans spending a lot more than they report in income). And you can find out much more relevant things about true deprivation and degradation by focusing on long-term AFDC dependency than you can by using Molly Orshansky's poverty line.

Or to take another example, we should quit measuring education inputs like spending, class size, and even high school graduation rates, and start measuring instead the relevant outputs — namely what exactly the students are capable of doing. Unfortunately, the studies and polemics from the Children's Defense Fund, and the Child Welfare League, and the Food Research and

FIGURE 1. CHILDREN w/MOTHERS < H.S. GRADUATE
ADOLESCENTS 10–14

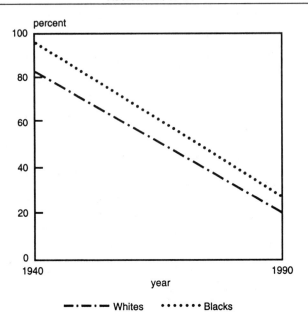

Source: "Changing Families and Adolescents
in the Post-War Years," Gretchen Cornwell,
David Eggebeen, Laurie Meschke

FIGURE 2. CHILDREN WITH 4 OR MORE SIBLINGS
ADOLESCENTS AGE 10–14, BY RACE

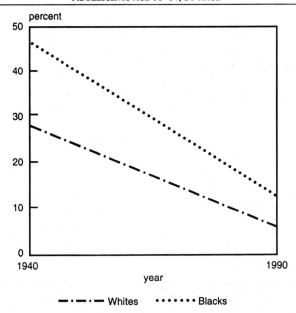

Source: "Changing Families and Adolescents
in the Post-War Years," Gretchen Cornwell,
David Eggebeen, Laurie Meschke

FIGURE 3. BIRTHS TO TEENAGERS

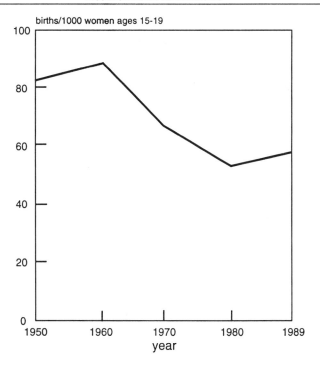

Source: U.S. National Center for
Health Statistics

FIGURE 4. BIRTHS TO TEENAGERS
LEGITIMATE AND ILLEGITIMATE

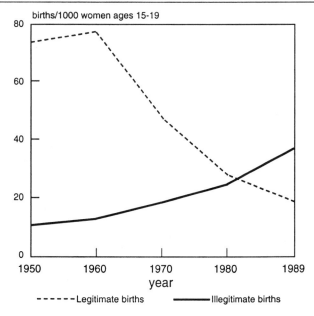

Source: U.S. National Center for
Health Statistics

18

FIGURE 5. INFANT MORTALITY RATES

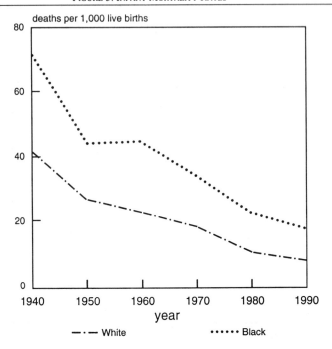

Source: U.S. National Center for
Health Statistics

FIGURE 6. LOW BIRTHWEIGHT RATES

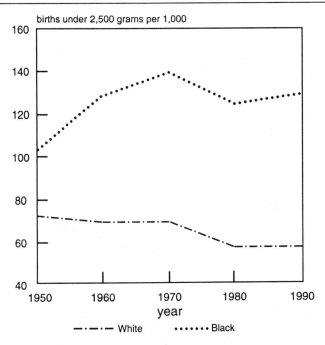

Source: U.S. National Center for
Health Statistics
Note: 1950 & 1960 - Black and other

Action Center, and other such places that dominate media headlines are still built around all the old measures: official poverty levels, teen births, infant mortality rates, and education spending. Too many academic studies make the same mistake, partly I think because of terrible fear that a focus on behavioral issues will be seen as "blaming the victims."

This is most unfortunate. Because the only alternative to a shift away from the old physical measures of family problems is what you might call well-documented stupidity. On many conventional measures, for instance, today's New York City public high school graduate is far better off than his 1950's counterpart. It is only when you factor in some softer measurements of behavior and context — like school violence rates, and sexual activity patterns, and abortion histories, and drug experience, and whether the child knows his or her father, and whether the father is married to the mother, and the visibility of employed persons in their neighborhood, and local homicide levels and weapons use — that you begin to recognize today's real problems. To strike a positive note let me point out that some data gatherers and data analyzers are beginning to make precisely the kind of efforts I am calling for. An excellent example is the detailed material on family structure and outcomes gathered by NCHS in the 1988 National Health Interview Survey on Child Health. Over the last couple years, Deborah Dawson of the NCHS has put out some very important

and accessible family status reports using this data. Likewise, Paul Ryscavage, Gordon Green, Edward Welniak, and John Coder of the Census Bureau have made some most useful studies of the effect of family type change on income levels and distribution. Our government data-gathering agencies have done a pretty good job of remaining current and relevant. Unfortunately, advocates, academics and policy makers haven't given excellent information of this type nearly the attention it deserves — I believe because they would rather not face some of the conclusions it would force on them.

One result of this blundering is that intelligent interpretation of our family problems increasingly comes from outside established channels, from small think tanks and independent researchers not wed to the old ways. The recent reports of the National Commission on America's Urban Families and Senator Rockefeller's National Commission on Children, for instance, were both built primarily on analyses from outside the old family-research mainstream.

I believe that those social scientists and policy makers who insist on clinging to the old and increasingly artificial poverty-war measurements of physical and material status, and resist examinations of personal character, attitudes and behaviors, are going to make themselves irrelevant to the process of understanding and then solving today's major family problems.

EDWARD L. SCHOR, M.D.
Associate Professor of Pediatrics and Community Medicine
Tufts University School of Medicine

Health, Health Behavior and Family Research

Families have important influences on the health, health beliefs, and health-related behaviors of individuals. The impact of families on health is especially apparent during childhood and adolescence, although it has lifelong consequences. In theory, intervening with families to maintain, improve, or promote health is an attractive strategy. However, reaching families for the purpose of changing their health beliefs and behaviors is not an easy task, and likely requires strategies that rely on a variety of social institutions in addition to the health care system. Effective interventions will require a much greater understanding of the health-related roles of families and of families' interactions with social institutions than now exists.

FAMILY STRUCTURE AND HEALTH

It is tempting to begin the study of the effect of families on health by focusing on structural characteristics of families. Underlying this approach to research is the belief that form influences function, that by knowing if a family has one parent rather than two, has experienced a divorce, or has a teenage rather than an older mother, one can draw conclusions about the likely health and well-being of the family's members.

A substantial amount of research has been done to examine the association between family structure and health. For example, marital status has been associated with mortality rates, and with preventive health behaviors of adults. Single-parenthood has been associated with poorer physical health status and socio-behavioral outcomes for children, and increased use of health care services for less serious health problems.

Similar to structural variables, family socio-demographic variables often are ascribed causal roles in the pathway to health. They have been found to correlate with measures of health and health behaviors, and health status increases with each higher level of social class.

Much previous family health research has focused on structural and socio-demographic characteristics of the family. The limitations of this focus are worth highlighting. First, these two categories of data are not mutually independent; family structure is related to social class. For example, the adverse health and health risk behaviors of female-headed households seem more related to the relative poverty of these households and to the lack of social support than to the single parent status of the mother.

Secondly, neither family structure nor socio-economic status indicators are necessarily useful explanatory variables. For example, while children of divorced parents seem to have a higher rate of emotional problems, this diminished health status seems unrelated either to living with a single parent or to the diminished economic resources of their divorced family. Rather, it seems to be due to the pre-divorce conflict within the home and to either the internalization of blame or the separation and loss they experience. Thus, to draw conclusions based solely on such variables as household composition, marital status, or social class indicators reflects an overly simple concept of how families function within the realm of health and disregards other important aspects of family life. Rather than limiting studies of family health to elements of structure, research should be directed toward understanding the underlying mechanisms by which structural and socio-demographic characteristics of families exert an effect on family health. What aspects of family health research are most likely to be productive?

HEALTH BELIEFS AND HEALTH PROMOTING AND HEALTH RISK BEHAVIORS

Families have been shown to influence health care utilization. They also are likely to influence the onset or course of some health problems, particularly those that can be forestalled, or entirely prevented, or which are manifest by deterioration of functional health status and well-being. Thus, the influence of families is most likely to be found in the development of health beliefs, health care seeking behaviors, and in the adoption of both health risk and health promoting behaviors.

How and to what extent do families influence the development of health beliefs and behaviors? Figure 1 is a useful schema for isolating some important elements in this process.

First, it is important to acknowledge that the processes illustrated in Figure 1 occur within a historical, cultural, and socio-economic context. The figure illustrates a hypothetical relationship among a number of factors that may influence individual health beliefs and behaviors during childhood and adolescence. For the sake of discussion the number of factors considered have been limited to three, (1) the family, (2) the peer group, and (3) the other proximal influences of a complex of community, schools, and media. If this model were applied to adults, the peer group and proximal influences would be more broadly defined to include colleagues and work site respectively.

These three sectors operate on a pre-existing and developing biological and psychological template. This template incorporates innate characteristics that include individual resilience and vulnerability to physical, social, and psychological stresses.

A Point In Time: Among the three factors represented in Figure 1, families are virtually the sole influence on health during infancy, and the predominant influence for many years. Over time the influence of families diminishes while the

FIGURE 1. CONTRIBUTORS TO CHILD HEALTH PROMOTING AND HEALTH RISK BEHAVIORS

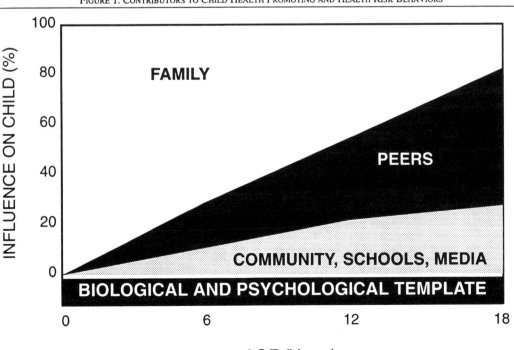

TABLE 1
Functions of the Family

INSTRUMENTAL FUNCTIONS	COGNITIVE/AFFECTIVE FUNCTIONS

Families provide...
   Food
   Clothing
   Shelter
   Safety
   Supervision
   Hygiene
   Health Care
   Education
	Families provide . . .
	   • Social Support
	     Cared For & Loved
	     Valued/Esteemed
	     Communication
	     Shared Values
	     Companionship
	   • Socialization
	     Transmit Values
	     Connection to World
	   • Education
	     Coping Skills
	     Life Skills

influences of peer groups and the community complex increase. If, for example, Figure 1 was used to show a cross-sectional representation of the factors accounting for alcohol use by 18 year old adolescents, roughly 20% of the variance of that health risk behavior would be accounted for by family factors, 50% by peers, and 30% by the community complex including community values, access to alcohol, exposure to media that promote drinking, and so on. Someone planning an intervention at this age would seem to be well advised to focus on peer and community influences.

Despite the acknowledged importance of the family to health, the mechanisms by which families influence the life experiences of their members and thus their health beliefs and behaviors remain to be elucidated and quantified. (Table 1 lists possible mechanisms by which families influence the health and well-being of their members.)

The same can be said for other influential sectors. Certainly, those health behaviors that are routine, valued, and an ever present part of an individual's culture are most likely to be adopted. Frequently omitted from research on the impact of family on individual health are issues of the duration of exposure to the influence, the degree of intensity of the influence, when in the life cycle the exposure occurred, and the interval between the event and measurement of the health outcome.

It should be noted that the relative contributions of each sector, (e.g., family, peers, and community) depicted in Figure 1 are hypothetical. In few, if any, cases do we know what is the relative contribution of each sector to health beliefs or behaviors. A first task awaiting family health researchers is to gather the data that would allow accurate rendi-

tions to be drawn of age-specific cross-sectional maps for alcohol use and other health risk behaviors. I suspect that were the data available, the graph would look somewhat different for different categories of health belief, and of disease preventing, health promoting, or health risk behaviors. Consequently, interventions with families would have to be specific to each behavior.

Cumulative Experience: While most previous family health research has been cross-sectional, Figure 1 depicts a longitudinal process. An obvious message of this graph then is that health at any age has a history of preceding influences and experiences. While the drinking behavior of an eighteen year old may at eighteen appear to be influenced only 20% by the family, the family's actual cumulative contribution to that behavior might be closer to 60% over the preceding 18 years. Taking into account this longitudinal influence of the family, the graph would look considerably different for other health behaviors. For example, tooth-brushing patterns may be established by an early age; subsequent family influence would be negligible, and the slope of the graph would become flat.

Clearly, age of the child is an important factor in determining the relative influence of family, friends, and community. Having data to create accurate models of the influence of families over the life cycle for each health behavior would be extremely useful to guide the timing of intervention strategies.

Interactions: The lines dividing the sectors illustrated on the graph are deceptively and erroneously solid. The sectors do not operate independently; each sector influences and is influenced by the other. For example, where and with whom children spend their time is to a great extent influenced by their families. Families in other ways influence the content of their child's experience. Some of the influence of families is no doubt exerted directly, in real time, through restrictions on exposure to external factors. Families also exert their influence by establishing and conveying values and norms for behavior and thereby buffering the effect of those factors such as peers and community. A family's participation in other influential settings such as schools, has been shown to have important effects on outcomes. No doubt there are numerous other mechanisms by which families interact with other sources of influence. These mechanisms need to be identified and measured. The interfaces between sectors are extremely important locations at which to intervene to modify family health behaviors.

Transitions: Figure 1 also demonstrates that the relative impact of the family, peers, and the community are likely to change rather dramatically at certain critical periods. For example, usually, entry into elementary school, leaving home for college or independent living, and marriage all signal important changes in the relationships and relative influence of the family. These transitions may not only represent times of change in the relative influence of each sector, but also may provide special opportunities to intervene to affect health. Decisions made at particular points in the life cycle can affect later health pathways. Sexual activity postponed, dietary habits established, or dental care obtained can have lifelong consequences. A better understanding of the primary influences on health at each age and transition would allow better targeting of interventions be they clinical, educational, or social.

Structure and Function: In addition to transitional events, there are a number of other family events that alter family structure and influence health

and health behaviors. Marriage, divorce, and remarriage are likely to change with whom children have contact and thus from whom they learn. Other circumstances such as single-parenthood and two-parent working families may place children in out-of-home care settings that can increase the likelihood of infectious disease or injury, and provide alternative models of health behaviors. There is much to be learned about the effects of various family structures on the emotional and social functioning and physical health of children. Figure 1 could be extended to represent the influence of family over the life course. There is evidence that both marriage and parenthood, as well as other events such as death of a spouse which cause structural changes in the family, have significant effects on health and health behaviors of adults. These associations need further study.

SUMMARY

There is some, although insufficient, understanding of how each sector, especially the family sector, operates to influence the health and health behaviors of its members. Some areas for exploration include: the relative contribution of families at each age or developmental stage for important health promoting and health risk behaviors; the cumulative and lingering influence of families on these behaviors over the life course; critical points in the life course when the balance of influence shifts; the mechanisms by which families shape and influence health beliefs and behaviors; how families interact with and modify or buffer the influence of other factors in the life experience of individuals; and the relationship between the family and an individual's innate biological and psychological characteristics of vulnerability and resilience. Finally, by understanding how family structure and social class alter the health-related functions of families, one mechanism of their effect will be better understood.

JAMES S. HOUSE, PH.D.
Department of Sociology and
Survey Research Center
The University of Michigan

The Political Economy of Families and Health:

Comments in Response to a Paper by

Frances Goldscheider

Our nation is entering into a critical period of debate, and hopefully action, regarding social and economic policy and health and health care policy. Both debates are very important in their own right, but what is less appreciated is that they have important implications for each other. President Clinton and others have emphasized that reforming our medical care system is crucial not only to assuring greater equity and access to health care but also to stemming a still growing drain on the public and private sectors of our economy.

Less recognized at this point, I think, is that social and economic factors and policy are major determinants of health, arguably more important at this time than many or most aspects of health care. An increased focus on preventive and primary care can have a major impact on health and life expectancy, especially for children and women of child-bearing age. This has clearly been shown in selected undeveloped countries, though we have yet to fully apply the lessons of their example (Rockefeller Foundation, 1985). However, neither advances in medical technology nor changes toward universal health care or health insurance systems in most developed countries can be shown to have had major impacts in

recent years on health and life expectancy, especially in adulthood.

This has been strikingly evident in the persistence of socioeconomic differentials in health and life expectancy in many developed countries throughout this century. Data from Canada, shown in Figure 1, are instructive in this regard.

They show large socioeconomic differentials in mortality at most ages in 1971 before the advent of national health insurance. And, with the exception of female infant and child mortality, these differentials had not diminished by 1986, almost a decade after the inception of the Canadian national health insurance system (Wilkins, Adams & Brancker, 1989). Also worth noting in these data is that the socioeconomic mortality differentials are greatest in infancy and early childhood and again in middle adulthood, but are substantially diminished in adolescence and early adulthood and again in older age. Available data from the United States and United Kingdom are generally consistent with these trends (see House et al., 1990). Looked at in another way, higher socioeconomic strata in our and other developed societies are arguably experiencing levels of health and life expectancy that are increasingly as good as may be currently biologically possible, as

Figure 1. Relative Mortality (Q5/Q1)*
Urban Canada, 1971–1986

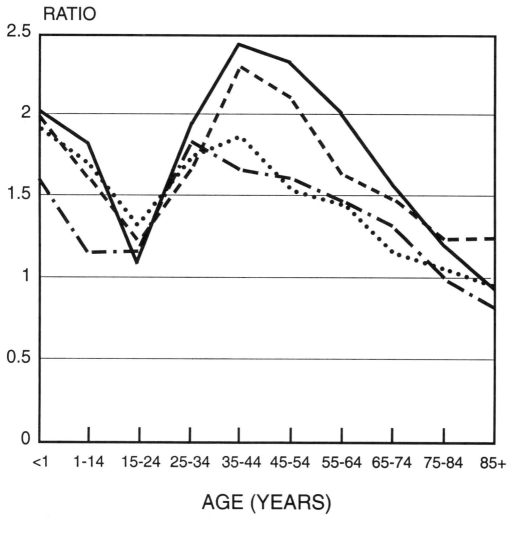

RATIO

AGE (YEARS)

– – – Males 1971 ——— Males 1986
• • • • • Females 1971 — • — Females 1986

*Q5 = Poorest neighborhoods
 Q1 = Least poor neighborhoods

Source: Statistics Canada/Health and Welfare Canada
(Wilkins, Adams & Brancker, 1989)

26

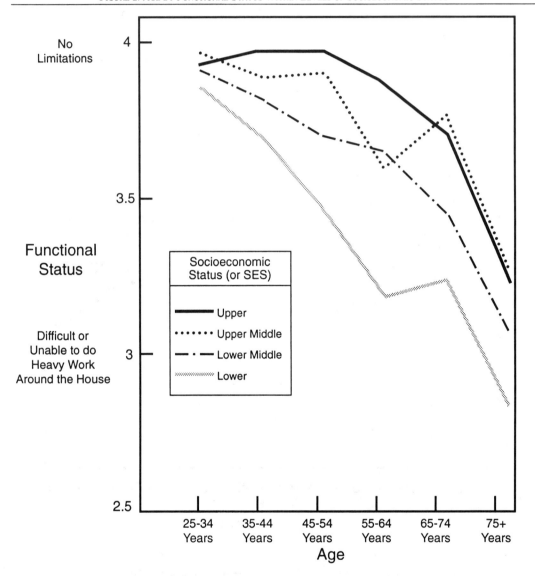

Source: House, et al. (1990). 1986 Americans' Changing Lives Interviews Survey data, n = 3,617
(adapted from House, et al., 1990)

evident in data from some of our current research, shown in Figure 2 (from House et al., 1990).

However, there is a great opportunity to prevent disease and to promote health and life expectancy at lower socioeconomic levels.

There are several important implications of these data. First, the greatest potential for preventing disease and promoting health in our society is concentrated at lower socioeconomic levels and among infants and children and adults of working age, and hence among the families of which they are a part. Second, as the level and distribution of medical care seems to be becoming less important as a determinant of health, our emphasis has shifted toward preventive approaches to promoting health and preventing disease (DHHS, 1990). Over the last several decades we have come to recognize that this involves reducing risky health behaviors and promoting healthful ones in areas like smoking, drinking, eating, seat belt use, etc. It also involves reducing exposure both to physical chemical biological hazards in the environment and to more recently recognized psychosocial risk factors such as chronic and acute stress, lack of social relationships and supports, and lack of control, efficacy or mastery over one's life (see House et al., 1990). Third, the family is a major determinant of health. That is, the nature, structure and functioning of families is a crucial determinant not only of patterns of illness behavior and health care utilization, which Dr. Schor and others have discussed, but also of health behaviors and the exposure to and experience of psychosocial risk factors such as stress, social relationships and supports, and sense of control or efficacy (Ross, Mirowsky, & Goldscheider, 1990). Finally, it is crucial to recognize that the nature, structure, and functioning of families, and hence the families' influence on health, is shaped by the larger macrosocial and economic context in which they are embedded.

Dr. Goldscheider has highlighted several major trends in the nature of families in the U.S., and suggested their implications for health. Her observation of the rise of joint survivorship indicates that health, here the growth of life expectancy, also has important effects on the family. Joint survivorship may in turn affect health through its impact on intergenerational patterns of social relationships, social support, and caregiving.

Given the limits of time and my expertise, I will pass on, as Dr. Goldscheider has, to several other interrelated changes in the nature, structure and functioning of families, which are very consequential for understanding the impact of the family on health, and some of the variations in health by age and socioeconomic status evident in Figures 1 and 2. First is the increase in marital disruption via divorce. Second is the rise in single-parent families due to divorces and to the rise in births to unmarried women. And third is the increase in individuals living alone, which stems, as Goldscheider notes, in part from the decline in two-parent families and also from changes in the values and options regarding living arrangements for unmarried persons, both young and old.

There is growing evidence that each of these changes in patterns of family life may be deleterious for health, either directly or through other patterns of social behavior to which they are linked. Both divorce and widowhood are among those negative life events that have been found on average to deleteriously affect physical and mental health. However, whether there are negative effects in a particular case, and how serious they are, depends on the nature of the individuals involved, their prior marital relationships, and the social and economic supports available to them. For example, the health of men seems to be more adversely affected than the health of women by being or becoming unmarried (House et al., 1988). As Goldscheider suggests, if this were more widely recognized, it might provide an incentive for men to become or stay married, while we also try to increase their incentives via greater involvement in parenting.

Two important sequelae of divorce and of unmarried parenthood are especially consequential for the health and well-being of both children and their single parents, especially women. First, divorce and being an unmarried parent greatly increases the risk of poverty or financial deprivation and stress, and these are powerful risk factors for deleterious physical and mental health outcomes for all members of a family (Ross et al., 1990). Second, even beyond the financial stress and deprivations, single parent families are in other ways stressful for both the parents and the children. Having only one adult to cope with the demands facing any family, is likely to leave both that parent and her or his children feeling overstressed and undersupported. Children are a strain on the mental health of all parents, but especially unmarried mothers (Mirowsky & Ross, 1989). A growing body of research of McLanahan (1989) and others suggests that children in single parent families are at increased risk for a wide range of adverse outcomes in terms of school performance, socioeconomic attainments and subsequent family formation, as well as physical and mental health. It should be recognized, as Dr. Goldscheider suggests, that the mere presence of a second parent is not a panacea for these problems. Indeed Mirowsky and Ross (1989) show that women who work and have childcare problems but whose husbands are not helpful with these problems, are at very high risk of psychological distress. In fact, both working and having children are likely to be beneficial to the health of women and men if they have support from each other and the external environment in managing their multiple roles. These are the kinds of families which Dr. Goldscheider rightly urges us to promote.

The dramatic increase in adults living alone that Dr. Goldscheider documents must also be attended to. The evidence that living alone per se is risky or deleterious for health is less conclusive, however, and more and better research is needed

(Hughes & Gove, 1981). However, individuals living alone are prone to be more socially isolated and financially deprived, both of which are clearly risk factors for physical and mental health (House et al., 1988). Even if living alone per se is not risky, efforts must be made to ensure that the potential social isolation and financial deprivation often associated with it are compensated for or buffered in other ways.

In sum, what we know about the health effects and risks of the nature, structure, and functioning of families largely supports Dr. Goldscheider's argument that we cannot view neutrally the dramatic increases in divorce, single parenthood, and living alone of the last several decades. And I am sympathetic to Dr. Goldscheider's desire to reverse "the growth in non-family living" and promote the formation and stability of marriages and intact families. I am less certain that we agree on the extent to which this is possible and desirable, or the routes through which it might occur. She speaks only briefly to these issues, focusing on promoting greater and more equal involvement of men in both household work and parenting, and on reducing normative pressures for "independent living" of unmarried older and younger adults. How we do this is unclear.

To return to my opening theme, I would emphasize that it is very important that we increasingly recognize the reciprocal relations between family and health, but it is equally important that we recognize that health, families and the relations between them are shaped by broader social and economic factors and policies. The rise in women's labor force participation, in divorce and single parenting, and in living alone reflect social and economic trends which have pushed as well as pulled women into the labor forces, increased the political and economic autonomy and equity of women, and made the single person households both more necessary, more possible, and more desired. We can do things socially, legally, and politically that will make possible more and better family life. If both women and men are able to increase their hourly earnings, and have access to policies and programs which facilitate both childcare and the parents' involvement in parenting, they are more likely to be better spouses for each other and better parents for their children. Thus, promoting greater growth and equality in wages and income, as well as increasing public and private support for child and elder care, parenting and intergenerational caretaking, are all major avenues to increasing the health and

longevity of both families, and the parents, children and elders which comprise them.

However, we also need to recognize that the social and cultural forces which have increased marital instability, single parenting, and independent living cannot, and should not, be totally transcended. Thus, we must seek to understand not only how we might slow or counteract the trends toward increasing marital instability, single parenting, and living alone, but also how we can create social and economic conditions and policies which will allow people to make these choices, as they will or even must, but will also mitigate or eliminate adverse effects on their health. Were divorced or single parents and their children better able to avoid extremes of economic deprivation, to maintain pre-existing social relationships with friends, relatives, schools, employees, and community organizations, and to have more adequate supports for child care and their own involvement in parenting, the deleterious health effects of divorce and single parenthood on parents and children might be substantially reduced, if not eliminated. Similarly, research suggests that maintaining and supporting the economic viability and social integration of single person households can mitigate or eliminate adverse health effects of living alone (Hughes & Gove, 1981).

How to both maintain and promote the health of more traditional families and their members and also the health of new forms of households or families and their members is a challenge for both research and policy. The last decade has seen a substantial growth in research on families and health (Ross et al., 1990). But much remains to be learned, especially about the longer term health effects of family and household arrangements which are relatively new, at least on a widespread scale, and about conditions which can exacerbate or alleviate potential adverse health effects of such new family and household forms, as well as of distressed or disturbed traditional families and relationships. We also need to understand more about the role of broader social and economic forces in affecting families and health and the relations between them, so that social and economic trends and policies can be better formulated or evaluated for their impact on health and on families, much as we now consider the economic or environmental impact of such policies and trends. We cannot understand or improve families or health without better understanding and improving the social and economic phenomena and policies that shape the nature of families and health, and the relations between them.

REFERENCES

DHHS (1990). *Healthy people 2000: National health promotion and disease prevention objectives: Summary.* Washington, DC: Department of Health and Human Services.

House, J. S., Landis, K., & Umberson, D. (1988). Social relationships and health. *Science, 241,* 540-545.

House, J. S., Kessler, R. C., Herzog, A. R., Mero, R. P., Kinney, A. M., & Breslow, M. J. (1990). Age, socioeconomic status, and health. *The Milbank Quarterly* 68(3):383-411.

Hughes, M. M., & Gove, W. R. (1981). Living alone, social integration, and mental health. *American Journal of Sociology, 87*:48-74.

McLanahan, S. (1989). *The two faces of divorce: Women's and children's interests.* Paper presented at the Annual Meeting of the American Sociological Association, 1989.

Mirowsky, J., & Ross, C. E. (1989). *Social Causes of Psychological Distress.* New York: Aldine-de-Gruyter.

Rockefeller Foundation. (1985). *Good health at low cost.* New York: Rockefeller Foundation.

Ross, C. E., Mirowsky, J., & Goldscheider, K. (1990). The impact of the family on health: The decade in review. *Journal of Marriage and the Family, 52,* 1059-1078.

Wilkins, R., Adams, O., & Brancker, A. (1989). Changes in mortality by income in urban Canada from 1971 to 1986. *Health Reports, 1*(2):137-174.

BRENT C. MILLER, PH.D.
Professor
Department of Family & Human Development
Utah State University

Summary

In summary, the major premise of Dr. Goldscheider's paper was an increasing life span has brought with it joint survivorship which significantly changes family relationships, especially between parents and children and between spouses. Further, single parenting, divorce, and remarriage all create economic disadvantages for children. The emergence of non-family living has likewise created financial hardships, but moreover, is related to poor health and quality of life. In conclusion, the keynote address suggests the reintegration of men into parenting would produce more rewarding family life as would the reintegration of the generations.

Dr. Schor's response paper highlighted the limitation of using socio-demographic variables to analyze the family, since they are not independent of one another and cannot be used as causal indicators. The paper stressed the family's influence in establishing health beliefs, health care seeking behaviors, and the adoption of health risk and health promotion behaviors. Dr. House's presentation also noted the family's important role in health promotion and preventive behaviors. Further, Dr. House postulates that even though made by choice, family changes such as divorce, single parenthood, and singlehood are deleterious to health, and policy decisions must be reformulated to target new family concerns.

Finally, Dr. Zinsmeister's paper suggested that the safest and healthiest environment for children is within the natural, intact family. He believes there is a need to more accurately measure behavioral indicators.

Dr. Goldscheider defended her position that family relationships will not improve until we redefine "family" to reflect recent demographic changes. She suggests it is the commitment of the family members to each other within the unit that defines the relationship, not the traditional or non-traditional structural aspects. Dr. Goldscheider feels policies should reinforce the duration of the commitment itself versus addressing the family based on its legal definition. She and other panelists voiced their concerns regarding the lack of data on fathers' roles in the family.

Dr. Kris Moore of Child Trends noted current data collection methods are based on a household orientation which does not reflect non-family relationships within a household. This has become more of an issue with the dramatic increase of persons living in non-traditional family settings. She further noted that there is a need for databases to integrate socio-demographic variables so that researchers can better measure family processes that affect health. This would include race and ethnicity and psychological and socioeconomic structures of families.

Federal statistics have a restrictive definition of a family. Dr. Mary Grace Kovar from the National Center for Health Statistics explained that the Census Bureau identifies families as people related by blood, marriage, or adoption who live in the same household and share a common

30

entrance and common cooking facilities. This is an important consideration when trying to improve family statistics for health policy purposes.

The process by which people choose to enter different types of families must also be considered. Dr. Chris Bacharach from the National Institutes for Child Health and Human Development noted that these decisions are all affected by the larger social structures in which people live. Data sets must somehow reflect these pre-existing factors. Other panelists made similar comments regarding structural influences on the family.

The issues are overwhelming in terms of the types of data needed to study families. How can we make the federal data collection effort even marginally better to meet our needs? How can we take some of what we have and make it better? How do you capture family dynamics and family quality in a few survey questions, remaining cognizant of time and money constraints? As Dr. Felicia LeClere from the National Center for Health Statistics pointed out, large federal surveys can give certain types of family-based data but some of the qualitative work must still be based on smaller data collection efforts.

Drs. Manning Feinleib from the National Center for Health Statistics and David Olson from the University of Minnesota both underscored the importance and difficulties in measuring family dynamics. What makes certain families succeed while others fail? Of particular interest are cohesion and conflict within the family.

NICHOLAS ZILL, PH.D.
Westat, Inc.

A Family-Based Approach to

Analyzing Social Problems

The family is a basic building block of American society, fulfilling a variety of important functions for the young, the elderly, and those in the middle years of life. Over the last three decades, living arrangements and behavior patterns have changed so rapidly that many people are concerned about whether the family as we know it is "falling apart." This concern has led to a widespread desire for trustworthy information about what is really happening to families. It has also stimulated numerous studies aimed at discovering the effects that changing family norms are having on the performance of adults, the development of children, and the operation of other social institutions.

A guide to national surveys and other databases that can provide information about modern family life in the United States is now available (Zill & Daly, 1993). It was prepared by Margaret Daly, Christine Winquist Nord, and myself at Westat, and by Kristin Moore, Donna Ruane Morrison, Mary Jo Coiro, Bret Brown, Barbara Sugland, Nancy Snyder, and Connie Blumenthal at Child Trends. The guide describes the extensive body of survey and statistical data, much of it collected at public expense, that can help to answer common questions about American families and illuminate issues about the causes and consequences of family change. These databases have not been analyzed to produce anything like the wealth of facts, insights, and hypothesis tests that they could potentially yield. A major purpose of this guide is to encourage more researchers to take advantage of the rich set of databases that have been generated in the last 20 years.

The guide can also be of use to those who have no intention of carrying out analytic studies themselves, but want the best available answers to pressing questions about family trends. The guide catalogs the data resources that are potentially available to answer such questions, lists articles that have made use of major data sets, and gives names, addresses, and phone numbers of knowledgeable persons who can provide additional information on each database.

The production of the guide was sponsored by the Office of the Assistant Secretary for Planning and Evaluation of the U.S. Department of Health and Human Services. In underwriting the guide, that agency hoped to encourage more analysts to pursue a family-based approach to the formulation and appraisal of health and welfare policies. The next section of this paper describes what such an approach entails and why it might be fruitful.

A FAMILY-BASED APPROACH TO SOCIAL POLICY

Understanding what families are like and how they function in contemporary society can provide insights into a variety of social problems, including educational failure, unemployment, poverty, welfare dependence, domestic violence, delinquency and crime, mental illness, substance abuse, and other forms of health-damaging behavior. There are several reasons why a family-based approach to the analysis of social problems may be more productive than an individual-based approach. First of all, most people live in families. Even in our era of family breakdown and rampant individualism, this is still true. Thus, if it does nothing else, a family-based approach helps us understand the context of people's lives.

Second, dynamics within families have a great influence on the well-being and functioning of individual members. Quality-of-life surveys have repeatedly shown that a person's sense of how well his or her family life is going is closely linked to overall life satisfaction. A growing body of evidence indicates that a person's family situation is also an important determinant of job performance, financial well-being, effectiveness as a parent, crime victimization, and even physical health.

Third, social ills are not randomly distributed across families. Some families experience multiple problems, whereas other families are relatively problem free. Factors that lead to the development of one type of malady, such as frequent unemployment, often lead to others — such as family violence or health-damaging behavior.

Despite their problems, families usually carry out functions like rearing children and caring for frail or disabled adults more effectively and inexpensively than bureaucracies do. When families fail to perform certain functions or perform them badly, it makes sense for social agencies to seek ways to help the families do a better job. Only after these efforts have proven ineffective should thought be given to replacing the family. In this way, a family-based approach may make social programs more cost-effective.

For all of these reasons, many policy makers and service providers have been advocating a shift away from the categorical and individual-oriented programs that have dominated health, education, and welfare policies in the United States. What they propose instead are more integrated and family-centered schemes for delivering services. In order to develop such schemes, new kinds of data and analyses are needed.

DATA IMPLICATIONS OF A FAMILY-BASED APPROACH

The first requirement of a family-based approach is to know how many and what kinds of families are affected by a particular social problem. For example, how many families have experienced a crime victimization in the last year? How many have one or more members who suffer from a chronic mental illness? Conventional tabulations based on individuals provide little indication of the number of families that are touched by a disease or social malady. Nor do the usual analyses tell us much about the social and economic characteristics of the affected families.

A family-based approach also requires tabulation of data on the receipt of specific services with the family as the unit of analysis. Beyond this, information is needed on the problem "clusters" that families experience and the benefits "packages" they receive. These can lead to better appraisals of the adequacy of existing programs and delivery systems. Needed as well are data on the direct provision of care by family members, how much they pay for care provided by others, and the ways in which family members act as agents or intermediaries between the affected individual and health care or social service agencies.

Although some of these data elements are not available currently, many of them are. They are contained in existing survey archives, but appropriate family-level analyses have never been carried out. We hope that the existence of the guide may assist researchers in pursuing family-oriented analyses of a variety of social problems.

ANALYZING LINKS BETWEEN THE FAMILY AND THE INDIVIDUAL

In addition to family-based tabulations of problem occurrence and service receipt, the databases described in the guide can be used to analyze links between family situations and the functioning and well-being of individuals. These analyses can look at the effects of family circumstances on individual well-being, or look at the impact of individual behavior on the functioning of the family. Taking one tack, the researcher can examine whether being in particular family situations enhances or detracts from the performance or well-being of individual family members. For example, do married men who live with their wives and children tend to work more hours to support their families than separated, divorced, or never married men of the same age and educational background? Are children from divorced families more likely to drop out of high school than children from stable two-parent families?

Taking the opposite tack, the researcher can examine whether the behavior or health of individual members has favorable or unfavorable consequences for the functioning of their families. For example, are mothers who suffer from depression less likely to read to their young children regularly or play with them in intellectually stimulating ways? Are couples who have a retarded child more likely to become divorced than comparable couples who do not have such a child?

On either tack, when significant associations between individual behavior and family functioning are found, researchers have to heed the old injunction not to confuse correlation with causality. For example, marital status and work effort may be related because men with a strong work ethic are more attractive as mates and hence more likely to get and stay married than men with less diligence. Since random experiments on family behavior are usually not possible, researchers have to seek ways of controlling statistically for confounding and selection bias. New econometric methods have recently become available to assist the researcher in this task.

DEFINING "THE FAMILY"

Most of the data sets described in the guide adopt a definition of "the family" that is similar to the standard Census Bureau definition. That is, "a family is a group of two persons or more . . . related by birth, marriage, or adoption and residing together." Some researchers may wish to use a different definition of family, such as one that includes men and women who are not formally wed but have lived together as if married for some period of time. Others may want to consider adults who live elsewhere but provide regular assistance or financial support as family members, or include gay or lesbian couples in their definition of family. Some data sets contain information that would allow for analyses based on alternative definitions of family, but others do not. Information is included in the database descriptions to assist researchers in determining whether or not such analyses are possible.

TYPES OF SURVEYS AND STATISTICAL DATA COVERED IN THE GUIDE

The body of the guide consists of descriptions of major survey and statistical databases that contain useful information about the characteristics, expe-

riences, and behaviors of American families. These can be used by researchers who wish to carry out a study of a particular issue to locate a suitable database. The surveys described deal with an assortment of substantive issues, including health, education, employment and unemployment, poverty, crime, family formation and dissolution, child development, and substance abuse. The surveys are similar in that most are federally funded and nearly all are based on large national data collections using true probability samples of the population. A probability sample means that all persons in the sampled universe have a known chance of being included in the study. If such a sample is properly implemented and reasonable cooperation obtained, the survey findings should be generalizable, within a margin of sampling error, to the population as a whole. Furthermore, the various subgroups in the sample should accurately reflect the diversity of the U.S. population.

Characteristics of families in specific geographical areas. Although the surveys described in the guide have samples that number in the thousands, most are not large enough to allow estimates at the local level, as for a particular city or county. Also, most have not been designed to yield estimates for specific states of the U.S. On the other hand, nearly all of the surveys yield valid estimates for different regions of the U.S., (e.g., the Northeast, Midwest, South, and West), and for urban, suburban, and rural areas within those regions.

Databases that permit one to assess the characteristics of families in specific states, cities, or counties, are the Decennial Census of the population and the Vital Statistics system. The latter includes:

- the birth registration system (from which natality statistics are derived);
- the death registration system (from which mortality statistics are extracted); and
- less comprehensive systems for registering marriages and divorces (which provide indicators of family formation and dissolution).

Trends in family living. In addition to the Decennial Census and the Vital Statistics system, a data collection program that all family researchers should be familiar with is the Current Population Survey (CPS). The CPS is an ongoing national survey that the Census Bureau conducts each month for the Bureau of Labor Statistics. It is the federal government's primary mechanism for measuring trends in employment and unemployment. The CPS is also a major source of trend information about the nation's families, including trends in the marital situations of adults, the living arrangements of children, and family poverty. Recurring supplements to the CPS focus on topics such as family income and benefit receipt, child support and alimony, fertility, and school enrollment.

Family transitions. Three longitudinal studies described in the guide provide fertile ground for studies of the causes and consequences of family transitions. They are the Panel Study of Income Dynamics (PSID); the National Longitudinal Surveys of Labor Market Experience, especially the National Longitudinal Survey of Youth (NLSY), sponsored by the Bureau of Labor Statistics; and the Survey of Income and Program Participation (SIPP). The last is a recurring panel survey, with each panel lasting a relatively short time (two and a half years)(see reference 2). Topical modules of the SIPP cover issues such as retrospective information about the families of origin of adults in the survey, non-parental care arrangements for children, child support, functional limitations and disabilities of family members, support for non-household members, and the financing of post-secondary education.

Family growth and family activity patterns. Two cross-sectional surveys described in the guide focus explicitly on family relationships and family processes. One is the National Survey of Family Growth (NSFG), a recurring federal survey on issues related to family planning, childbearing, and infertility. The other is the National Survey of Families and Households (NSFH), which covers a wide range of family-related topics, including communication patterns, childrearing practices, family activities, division of household chores and responsibilities, family decision-making, marital satisfaction, community involvement, and contact with relatives outside the household.

Child and youth development. Several of the studies profiled in the guide deal with families with children and contain data that make it possible to relate family structure and functioning to aspects of children's development and well-being. These surveys include the National Survey of Children (NSC), the National Commission on Children's Survey of Children and Parents, the National

Health Interview Surveys on Child Health (NHIS-CH), and the Child and Mother Data supplements to the National Longitudinal Survey of Youth (NLSY-CS).

Post-divorce family functioning. Two important subnational studies provide information on divorce, child custody, and post-divorce family functioning. They are the Stanford Child Custody and Adolescent Custody Studies and the Noncustodial Parents Survey. National surveys that contain extensive information on marital separation and its consequences include the NSFH, the NSC, the NHIS-CS, the SIPP, and the Child Support and Fertility supplements to the CPS.

Public opinion on family matters. A number of the data sets described in the guide contain information on public attitudes about family values, family behavior, and family policy and show how these attitudes have changed over time. Relevant surveys include the General Social Survey (GSS) and the Study of American Families, as well as polls done for the National Commission on Children, the NSFH, and the NSC. The Public Opinion Location Library can guide the researcher to privately-sponsored opinion polls that contain questions on specific family-related topics of interest. Trends in youthful attitudes about family matters are tracked in an annual survey of high school seniors, Monitoring the Future.

Health, education, crime and other specific topics. The principal source of national data on family expenditure patterns is the Consumer Expenditure Survey. In the years between censuses, data on the housing of American families is provided by the American Housing Survey. Major health surveys described in the guide include the National Health Interview Survey (NHIS), which is conducted annually; the National Health and Nutrition Examination Survey (NHANES), which includes direct measures of physiological and biochemical variables, as well as interview-based information; and the National Medical Expenditure Survey (NMES).

Data on an important set of health-related behaviors, namely smoking, alcohol consumption, and use of illicit drugs are obtained in the National Household Survey on Drug Abuse. Self-reports of smoking and substance abuse by high school students are obtained in the annual school-based survey, Monitoring the Future.

In the area of education, the major surveys covered include three National Education Longitudinal Surveys (NELS), the National Assessment of Educational Progress (NAEP), and the National Household Education Survey (NHES), a recently begun series of cross-sectional surveys. Both the NAEP and the NELS involve direct testing of the academic achievement of representative samples of American youth.

Information on crime from the victim's perspective is gathered in the National Crime Victimization Survey (NCVS). Information about the family circumstances and backgrounds of offenders is obtained in a series of periodic surveys of inmates of various correctional institutions, such as the Survey of Juveniles in Custody. Data on family violence are obtained in the National Surveys of Family Violence and the Study of the National Incidence and Prevalence of Child Abuse and Neglect.

Families with elderly members. There is a growing body of survey data on families containing elderly members. Examples are the 1984 Supplement on Aging to the National Health Interview Survey, and its follow-up, the Longitudinal Study of Aging; the NHANES I Epidemiological Follow-up Study; the National Long Term Care Survey (Stone & Kemper, 1990); and the Current Beneficiary Survey of Medicare Recipients. Due to time and space limitations, these surveys are not covered in the guide.

FORMAT OF DATABASE DESCRIPTIONS

For each survey or statistical program described in the guide, material is presented on the purpose of the effort, the sponsoring agency, and the design of the survey or other data gathering procedure. Design information includes who was covered in the survey universe, how large the sample was, how often the survey has been conducted, and what completion rate was achieved. The content of the survey instrument or data collection form is summarized by listing topics covered, especially those involving potential causes or consequences of family behavior.

In the "Limitations" section of each survey write-up, we have tried to alert the analyst to gaps and biases in the data, particularly those that may cause difficulties or lead to erroneous conclusions for family-based studies. The "Availability" section tells where and how to get the data files, and gives the name, address, and phone number of

one or more contact persons. The "Publications" section gives a short bibliography of exemplary articles and reports that have made use of the data set in question.

The last three pages of each database write-up consist of checklists that show what the survey questionnaire or data collection form provides in the way of descriptive material about the families covered in the sample. These checklists show the varieties of families that can be identified in the database and the sorts of family-related variables against which other variables (such as measures of the prevalence of various social problems) can be tabulated. This is critical information for the analyst who is deciding whether or not the database can be used to investigate a particular issue.

The first checklist is composed of items pertaining to family-level characteristics; i.e., those that apply to the family as a whole. The second consists of items describing the characteristics of adult family members, and the third, of items on the characteristics of children in the family. The following sections give illustrations of the specific items included in the checklists.

Family-level characteristics. These include attributes that relate to the composition, social status, geographic location, life cycle stage, and functioning of the family. Specific items include the following:

- family composition (What do we know about who is in the family? About how they relate to one another? Is there information about per-time household members? About family members who no longer live in the household? About relatives who live nearby, but not in the household?);
- socioeconomic variables (Can we determine the family income level, or whether the family is below the official poverty line? Do we know whether the family receives welfare payments or food stamps or other non-cash benefits? Can we tell whether a language other than English is spoken in the home?);
- geographic/community variables (Does the database indicate in which region, state, county or city, zip code or telephone area code the family resides? Is there coded data pertaining to neighborhood quality or the state of the local labor market at the time of the survey?);
- stage in the family life cycle (Do we know the age of the adult respondent or his or her

NHIS—1988 Child Health Supplement
Year of Questionnaire: 1988
Sample size: 17,110 children aged 0-17
FAMILY LEVEL CHARACTERISTICS

Family Composition
- Full roster of household members (first name, age, sex, and relationship to reference person of each member)
○ Partial roster of household members
- Number of adults in household
- Number of children in household
○ Approximate relationship of family members to householder, child, or one another
- Exact relationship of family members to householder, child, or one another
- Information about part-time household member[1]
○ Information about family members no longer living in household
○ Information about relatives who live nearby but not in household

Socioeconomic
- Total family income
○ Number of persons who depend on family income
○ Sources of income
○ Income amounts identified separately by source
- Poverty status
- Welfare status
○ Food Stamps receipt
○ Child support receipt
- Medicaid coverage
- Private health insurance
○ Home ownership/renters
○ Assets (other than home ownership)
○ Public housing status
- Telephone in household
○ Language other than English spoken in home

Geographic/Community Variables
- Region of country
○ State of residence
○ County/city/MSA of residence
- Size/type of community
○ Zip code
○ Telephone area code
- Metropolitan residence
○ Neighborhood quality
○ Local labor market

Stage in Family Life Cycle
- Age of adult respondent or spouse/partner
- Marital status of adult respondent or spouse/partner
- Employment status of adult respondent or spouse/partner
- Presence of own children in household[2]
- Age of youngest own child in household[2]
- Age of oldest own child in household[2]
- Existence of own children who have left home
○ Intention to have (more) children in future

Family Functioning
○ Family activities or time use
○ Community involvement (civic, religious, recreational)
○ Family communication patterns
○ Family decision-making
○ Marital conflict
○ Marital happiness/satisfaction
○ Parent-child conflict
○ History of marital separations
○ History of family violence
○ History of marital counselling

NOTES
1. Armed Services members.
2. Available if adult respondent is child's parent.

spouse/partner? Can we differentiate adults who were never married from those who were formerly married? Or those who have not yet had children from those who no longer have children living at home? Or those who are retired from those who are unemployed or not in the labor force for other reasons?); and

- family functioning (Does the database provide any information about family activities or time use patterns? About the family's level of community involvement? Do we know how much family members communicate with one another or how family decisions are made? Are there indicators of marital conflict or marital happiness or satisfaction? Do we know whether the family has a history of marital separations, family violence, or receipt of marital counseling?).

Two important distinctions relating to family composition are captured in the family-level checklists. The first involves whether or not a complete roster of household members is taken as part of the data collection procedure. A full roster means that one person in the household is defined as the reference person, and all household members are listed by age, sex, and relationship to the reference person.

The full roster is most useful from a family analysis perspective. It enables the analyst to derive information about family size, number of siblings, presence of extended relatives, and presence of non-related adults or children. However, some studies take only a partial roster of household members, or just collect summary information about the number of adults or the number of children in the household. When the roster is less complete, the analytic possibilities are obviously more constrained. Indeed, if no relationship information is collected, it may not even be possible to tell whether the household contains a family at all.

A second important distinction captured in the checklist is whether relationships between family members have been captured in exact terms or approximate terms. Exact relationships mean, for example, that when a person is described as a child's mother, the interviewer probes to find out whether the mother is the child's birth mother, adoptive mother, stepmother, foster mother, or other female guardian. Likewise for the child's father. Sibling relationships are similarly specified as to whether, for example, two brothers are full brothers, half brothers, adoptive brothers, or stepbrothers.

It is only when family relationships have been determined exactly that it becomes possible to identify stepfamilies, or "blended" families, or adoptive families, and carry out separate or comparative analyses of these family forms. In addition, specification of exact relationships opens up possibilities for behavior genetic analyses that try to separate family environmental influences from genetic influences on children's development, learning, and behavior.

Characteristics of adult family members. In the checklist on adult characteristics, separate note is taken of the information provided about the focal adult or adult reference person, his or her current spouse who resides in the household, and a current or former spouse who did not live in the same household at the time of the survey. Typically, the most family-related information is obtained about the reference adult, considerably less about the resident spouse, and much less, if anything, about a former spouse or a current non-resident spouse.

Characteristics of child family members. In the checklist on child characteristics, information provided about a focal or reference child and information provided about other children in the family are separately coded. Even in surveys that focus on children or youth, it is often the case that much more information is obtained about the reference child than about other children in the family. This restricts analyses that seek to describe a family's children as a group, or that try to examine similarities or differences among different children in the same family. In some surveys, however, questions are asked about all children in a given age range. Alternatively, questions may be obtained about a random subset of children, such as two but no more. In these cases, relationships among family members can be analyzed.

I conclude this paper by discussing the advantages and drawbacks of using the large-scale data sets to study family circumstances and behavior. I also note some needed improvements in the collection of survey data on families, improvements that would make these data far more useful to researchers and policy analysts.

ADVANTAGES OF WORKING WITH LARGE-SCALE DATABASES

There are a number of advantages to be gained by carrying out a study of family behavior by means

CHARACTERISTICS OF ADULT FAMILY MEMBERS

Adult Respondent or Reference Person	Current Spouse in HH	Current or Former Spouse Not in HH	
●	●	○	Age
●	●	●	Gender
●	●	○	Race
●	●	○	Hispanic origin
○	○	○	Other origin/ethnicity
○	○	○	Religious affiliation
○	○	○	Religious participation
○	○	○	Country of birth
○	○	○	Immigrant status
○	○	○	English fluency
●	●	○	Current marital status
●	○	○	Marital history[2]
○	○	○	Cohabitation status
○	○	○	Cohabitation history
●	●	●	Parental status[3]
●	○	○	Number children ever born/sired[3]
●	○	○	Age at first birth[3]
○	○	○	Age of youngest child
●	○	○	Children living elsewhere
○	○	○	Duration at current address
○	○	○	Residential mobility
●	●	○	Educational attainment
○	○	○	Degrees attained
○	○	○	GED or regular HS diploma
●	●	○	Current enrollment
●	●	○	Current employment status
●	○	○	Hours usually worked (ft/pt)[3]
○	○	○	Weeks worked
○	○	○	Annual employment pattern
●	●	○	Main occupation
○	○	○	Earnings
○	○	○	Wage rate
○	○	○	Payment of child support
○	○	○	Aptitude or achievement score
●	●	○	Health/disability status
○	○	○	Self-esteem
○	○	○	Locus of control or efficacy
○	○	○	Depression or subjective well-being
○	○	○	Work-related attitudes

NOTES
2. Available if adult respondent is child's parent.
3. Available if adult respondent is child's mother.

of secondary analysis of a data set described in this guide as opposed to the collection and analysis of new data. The benefits include the following:

- The analysis of existing data usually takes far less time and costs less money than gathering and analyzing new data.
- The sample of families on which conclusions are based is likely to be larger and more representative of the general population.
- Sampling methods are explicitly defined and executed, and the completion rate achieved in the study is clearly specified. This is often not the case in university-based studies using small samples, volunteer samples, or samples of convenience.
- Information about demographic and socioeconomic characteristics of family members is gathered in well-established ways.
- Existing data sets can be used to study historical trends in family behavior and group differences in behavior at earlier points in time.
- Conclusions based on existing data sets may be less biased by demand characteristics that

CHARACTERISTICS OF CHILD FAMILY MEMBERS

Reference Child or Youth Respondent	Other Children (in HH)	
●	●	Age
●	●	Month and year of birth
●	●	Gender
●	●	Race
●	●	Hispanic origin
○	○	Other origin/ethnicity
○	○	Religious affiliation
○	○	Religious participation
○	○	Country of birth
○	○	Immigrant status
○	○	English fluency
●	○	Exact relationship to adult family members
●	○	Exact relationship to other children in HH
●	●	Marital status/history
○	○	Parental status/history
●	●	Current enrollment in regular school
●	○	Current enrollment in preschool/daycare
●	●	Highest grade completed
●	○	Grade now enrolled
○	○	Employment status/history
●	●	Health status
●	●	Handicapping conditions
●	○	Grade repetition
○	○	Aptitude or achievement score
●	○	Pregnancy/birth history
●	○	Psychological well-being
○	○	Delinquency

are often introduced when an investigator sets out to do a new survey on a specific topic, such as the effects of divorce on children.

The effort required to carry out secondary analysis studies has been significantly reduced. Many survey databases can now be obtained in well-organized and documented form from archives such as the Inter-University Consortium for Political and Social Research (ICPSR) at the University of Michigan and the Roper Center at the University of Connecticut. In 1992, the first archive of family studies on compact disk was produced by Sociometrics, Inc., with support from the National Institute of Child Health and Human Development. Nearly all of the data sets in the archive on a disk are described in the data guide.

DRAWBACKS OF USING EXISTING DATABASES

Although studying family behavior through analysis of existing data has distinct advantages, the researcher should also be aware of the limitations of the method. Among the drawbacks are the following:

- The majority of the data sets described in our volume do not contain the kinds of information that family researchers most want, especially measures of family process.
- A good deal of manipulation may be required to produce family-level information from survey files, which are typically organized with the individual respondent as the unit of data collection and analysis.
- Because of their individual orientation, many surveys lack appropriate weights for producing national estimates of the number of families (as opposed to the number of individuals) for whom a given characteristic applies.
- Rarely do the measures used in large-scale studies consist of single items or short scales, and some of the scales have low reliability or are not well-validated.

- Most of the behavioral measures contained in large-scale data sets are based on self-reports of survey respondents, which have inherent limitations and biases (see reference 4).
- Many data sets lack information that would permit the analyst to identify certain types of families, e.g., stepfamilies or families with adopted children.
- Even large databases usually contain relatively few cases of rare family types, and caution should be exercised in generalizing from these small sub samples.
- Because public-use data sets are widely available, but communication among users is imperfect, the analyst may unknowingly duplicate work that another researcher has already carried out. In other words, someone else may have gotten there first.

Balancing the Strengths and Weaknesses of Survey Data

There is a tendency for researchers who have not worked with survey data to take extreme positions on the value of such data. They either accept survey data in an uncritical fashion, or reject them out of hand as hopelessly biased and invalid. The truth is rather more complicated. Although survey measures are often blurred by both random noise and systematic bias, they almost always contain real "signal" as well. Experienced survey researchers can tease valid conclusions out of imperfect measures by looking at patterns of relationships rather than single numbers. Also, the imperfections of questionnaire-based measures have to be balanced against the virtues of large probability samples. These samples represent the full range of variation in attitudes, behaviors, and living arrangements, and include segments of the population that are often missing from small-scale studies based on samples of convenience.

Needed Improvements in Survey Data on Families

The process of reviewing and appraising the data sets described in the guide led the authors to develop definite ideas about the kinds of changes needed to make survey data on families more useful to both academic researchers and policy analysts. I conclude by presenting these recommendations in summary form.

First, the field of family research would benefit greatly if a standard set of family descriptors were used throughout the federal statistical system. This would make it possible, for example, to draw a more rounded picture of the health and well-being of specific types of families, of the problems they experience and the services they receive. By having uniform descriptors, information that is obtained in different surveys can be integrated at the subgroup level. The family-level checklist used in the guide illustrated the kinds of variables that ought to be contained in the standard set of descriptors.

Second, secondary research on families would be more fruitful if large-scale surveys made use of concepts and measures that matched the realities of modern family life. One of those realities is that in many of today's families, adults follow work schedules that enable them to balance work and family responsibilities. They do this by having one or both parents work only part-time, or for part of the year only, or on shifts that reduce the need for child care or enable one parent to be home when the children are home. Getting information about year-round work schedules and co-ordination of shifts between parents would yield a better understanding of the changing patterns of family life.

Another reality of modern life is that many families have members who live elsewhere but maintain contact with the family or provide financial support or assistance with child care. This member may be a separated or divorced parent, or a grandmother who lives in the neighborhood but not in the household. Surveys should collect more information about these non-resident family members and family interactions that cross household boundaries.

Family research would be aided if surveys obtained data on more than one family member at a time. This would make it possible, for example, to examine the influence of the health-related behavior of one spouse on the parallel behavior of the other. When, as is often the case, only one random adult per family is selected for study, such within-family effects cannot be analyzed.

Methodological research is needed to develop more accurate methods of assessing basic conditions of family living. Chief among these are indicators of the basic economic well-being of families. Current measures of family income suffer from substantial missing data and deliberate under-reporting of some forms of income because of fears that the respondent may be penalized by the government if she or he reports truthfully. Assessments of levels of living based on consumption or expenditure patterns (the goods and services available to the family) may prove more useful than assessments based on income.

Finally, family researchers could certainly make use of data sets that provided more information about how families are functioning as a unit. This means questions or observations about communication patterns and the division of chores and responsibilities within the family, on how family decisions are made, and how the family adjusts to changing economic circumstances and to developments in the education, work, and health situations of individual members. Obtaining valid data on these topics at reasonable cost may prove challenging; but federal agencies and private survey sponsors have to take on this challenge if we are to learn how family life is changing and find better ways of assisting families in carrying out their critical functions.

REFERENCES - NOTES

Zill, N., & Daly, M. (1993). *Researching the Family: A Guide to Survey and Statistical Data on U.S. Families.* Washington, DC: U.S. Department of Health and Human Services (also available from Child Trends, Inc., Washington, DC).

Current plans for the SIPP call for the duration of each panel to be extended to four years, beginning in 1995 or 1996.

Stone, R. I., & Kemper, P. (1990). Spouses of children and disabled elders: How large a constituency for long-term care reform? *The Milbank Quarterly, 67*(3-4), 485-5.

Some survey studies, such as the National Longitudinal Survey of Youth (NLSY) and the National Survey of Children (NSC), do not rely solely on self-report measures. They gather information from multiple informants and make use of other measurement methods, such as achievement testing of respondents or their children, or interviewer observation of the home environment and parent-child interaction.

John S. Lyons, Ph.D.
Rachel L. Anderson
Paul Brule
Sara Ellison
Sarah Walker
TGP, Inc.
and
Northwestern University Medical School

Systematic Review of the Peer-Reviewed; Scientific Literature on Family, Marital, and Community Variables Across Twenty Fields of Inquiry

This project was funded by the Department of Health and Human Services. The content of this paper does not necessarily represent the views of the U.S. government or the Department of Health and Human Services

INTRODUCTION

There is widespread agreement that the United States in the 1990s faces significant challenges in assisting families, marriages, and communities with the complex social difficulties in modern society. Divorce rates remain high; many families are headed by single parents; and communities face problems of violence and decay.

Policy initiatives at the federal, state, and local levels represent the best hope for beginning to address these problems. However, good policy requires input from a range of informed sources. Ineffective policy is likely to be created in an information vacuum.

Social science research represents a potentially important input into the policy debates surrounding these complex issues. However, if science is to effectively inform policy, strategies are needed that will allow for the synthesis of diverse findings across disparate fields of inquiry.

One strategy which potentially informs both social policy (the design of policy initiatives) and research policy (the identification of areas in need of further research development) is the systematic review. This is an empirical strategy of research synthesis that has an epidemiological approach to study either the field of research or a particular research question.

In order to begin a process of developing policy in the area of family, marriage, and the community, the Department of Health and Human Services, Division of Family and Long-term Care initiated a set of systematic reviews. The reviews were intended to accomplish the following objectives:

TABLE 1. FIELDS AND TOP-CITED JOURNALS SELECTED FOR SYSTEMATIC REVIEW.

Business
  Academic Management Review
  Administrative Science Quarterly
  Journal of Consumer Research

Child Development
  Child Psychology and Psychiatry
  Child Development
  Developmental Psychology

Clinical Psychology
  Journal of Abnormal Psychology
  Journal of Consulting and Clinical Psychology
  Health Psychology

Communications
  Communications Monographs
  Human Communication Research
  Public Opinion Quarterly

Economics
  Econometrica
  Quarterly Journal of Economics
  Journal of Political Economy

Education
  Harvard Educational Review
  American Educational Research Journal
  Reading Research Quarterly

Geriatrics
  Journal of the American Geriatric Society
  The Gerontologist

Health Services Research
  Medical Care
  Millbank Quarterly
  Health Services Research

Family and Marriage Research
  Journal of Marriage and the Family
  Family Relations
  Journal of Family Issues

Family and Marital Therapy
  American Journal of Family Therapy
  Family Process
  Journal of Marital and Family Therapy

Law
  Journal of Legal Studies
  Law and Human Behavior
  Law and Society Review

Medicine
  Journal of the American Medical Association
  New England Journal of Medicine

Political Science
  American Political Science Review
  Journal of Politics
  American Journal of Political Science

Psychiatry
  American Journal of Psychiatry
  Archives of General Psychiatry
  Hospital & Community Psychiatry

Public Health
  American Journal of Public Health
  Public Health Reports
  Journal of Health and Human Behavior

Rehabilitation
  Exceptional Children
  Journal of Learning Disabilities
  Learning Disability Quarterly

Sex
  Archives of Sexual Behavior
  Journal of Sex Research
  Journal of Sex and Marital Therapy

Sociology
  American Journal of Sociology
  Social Forces
  American Sociology Review

Substance Abuse
  Addictive Behaviors
  American Journal of Drug and Alcohol Abuse
  Journal of Studies on Alcohol

Urban Planning
  Urban Affairs Quarterly
  Journal of the American Planning Association
  Journal of Urban Economics

1. Determine the degree to which different fields of inquiry have studied family, marital, and community phenomenon;
2. Estimate the quality of this research effort;
3. Identify areas in which this research can be improved;
4. Synthesize the primary findings in each field with regard to the impact family, marital, and community variables have on the primary outcomes of interest to the selected fields.

In order to accomplish these goals, twenty different substantive fields of research inquiry were selected for review (see Table 1).

Systematic review techniques were then applied to the literatures. However, in order to un-

derstand the results of these reviews it is necessary first to understand the methodology used in this form of review.

SYSTEMATIC REVIEW STRATEGIES

There are currently three strategies that have been used to synthesize literature: traditional reviews, meta-analysis and systematic reviews. Traditional reviews have generally involved a guided discussion of the findings across a body of research. The main criticism of traditional reviews is that this technique is often subject to the biases (overt and covert) of the reviewer(s), and thus become commentary. This may be a problem in areas of controversy. For example, two recent traditional reviews on the psychosocial sequelae of abortion came to nearly opposite conclusions (Dagg, 1991 and Ney & Wickett, 1989). Part of this disparity resulted from the fact that less than 20% of the cited references appeared in both reviews.

Meta-analysis represented an important breakthrough in research synthesis in that it provided a means to statistically synthesize articles to test a particular hypothesis across a set of similar studies. Effect sizes are estimated from each identified study and then averaged across studies to determine a "literature-wide" effect size. Characteristics of the studies (e.g., quality of methods) can be used to predict these effect sizes to further understand the research. The major liability of meta-analysis is that it requires a body of research that tests the same research hypothesis. Thus, it is useful for identifying the effects of psychotherapy but not particularly useful as a technique to study research on a broad topic (e.g., religion in psychiatry).

Meta-analysis has been criticized because it is quite sensitive to issues regarding inclusion of articles into the averaging of effect sizes. Critics point to the problem of "adding apples and oranges" when combining studies with different hypotheses and designs. However, as Glass, McGaw and Smith (1981) have pointed out, adding apples and oranges can be quite useful when you are studying fruit. Therefore, systematic review techniques have evolved to allow for the compilation of methodological characteristics and findings across a broad field of inquiry. By carefully establishing reliable criteria for article inclusion and further defining a population of articles to sample, systematic review techniques can define the "state-of-the-art" in any given field of inquiry.

Systematic reviews have generally sampled research in peer-reviewed journal articles (Lyons et al., 1990; Larson et al., 1989, 1992). The peer-review process is the mechanism thought to best optimize the quality of research. Thus, articles published in peer-reviewed journals most likely represent the highest quality research. There are two general sampling strategies that can be used in accomplishing a systematic review: representative and exhaustive. Use of a representative sample identifies particular journals in a field (usually the most cited empirical journals) and a range of years. This defined population of articles is then thoroughly reviewed and each article is either included or excluded based on pre-determined criteria. For instance in the Larson et al., (1989) review of nursing home research, each article was reviewed for the inclusion of a sample of current

nursing home residents. Articles sampling nursing home populations were then reviewed in greater detail. Representative sample frames are well suited for defining the state-of-the-art in research methods or in determining whether a particular variable is well represented in a body of research (e.g., AIDS research, nursing home research in psychiatry).

Representative sampling in systematic review relies on peer-reviewed journal articles as the frame of reference. Such a strategy ignores potentially important research in books, book chapters, government documents, researchers' file drawers, and other places. However, the primary goal of the present systematic review is to provide a replicable synthesis of existing scientific state-of-the-art in specific fields of inquiry. Peer-reviewed journals offer two advantages over other media. First, the peer-review process represents a valuable (albeit flawed) mechanism of quality control. Research claims made in books and other documents are not necessarily required to undergo such a process. Therefore, it is reasonable to propose that the research presented in peer-reviewed journals is likely to be, on average, of higher quality. However, this does not mean that any given book chapter is of lower quality than any single peer-reviewed article.

Additionally, peer-reviewed journals offer some important advantages when the goal of the review is to study the nature of a field of inquiry. Articles from the topic peer-reviewed journals in a particular field can be assumed to represent that field. Often the topic journals in a field are sponsored by large national or international organizations that represent the field. Likewise, if journals are selected that are commonly cited by other authors in the field it can be assumed that these journals are the most influential.

These reasons for including only peer-reviewed journal articles by no means imply that important research is not contained in other places, they simply provide a rationale for defining a universe of information to be reviewed.

In sum, a systematic review treats individual studies like data or units of analysis, this is similar to the way a survey researcher treats each respondent. This 'disregard' for the individual study has led some to propose that both systematic reviews and survey research are insensitive to either the critical study or the special person. While this criticism is accurate, it is important to consider that as survey research does not replace the case study, systematic reviews do not replace in-depth discussions of single studies. The types of questions asked and the results obtained are merely different with these methods. So while a systematic review strategy does not implicitly value critical studies more than other studies on a related topic nor allow for detailed discussion of such, it can provide useful information in aggregate about a field of inquiry.

METHODOLOGY

Search Procedure. In order to accurately represent each of the twenty fields selected for review, the three general journals with the highest citation index rating were selected. Specialty journals within fields were excluded to maintain the representativeness of the review. In two fields, only two journals were selected as the next most cited journal was international and the remaining journals were specialties. Table 1 presents the twenty fields selected and the journals identified using the citation index Impact Factor.

The systematic review occurred in two steps. First, each article in each of these journals appearing from January 1, 1986 through December 31, 1990 was reviewed to determine whether or not the study was quantitative (included original data on at least one variable) and included a family, marital, or community variable.

Second, each identified quantitative article that included a family, marital, or community variable was reviewed on a number of the following dimensions:

Sample Characteristics—demographics
Methodological Characteristics—sample frame, design, etc.
Funding Source
Threats to Validity (Cook & Campbell, 1979)
Measures
Findings—for Family, Marital, and Community Variables

The form used to accomplish this second phase of the review can be found in the appendix of this report. To provide within field comparisons, 50 articles were randomly selected (using a random numbers table) from each field and reviewed in the first four dimensions listed above.

DEFINITIONS OF TERMS

In order to review family, marital, and community variables in these varying and complex litera-tures, it is necessary to first define (at least for present purposes) what is meant by these terms.

Marital variables refer to the measurement of any aspect of a person's status with regards to marriage. This definition not only includes marital status, per se, but also the measurement of the attitudes, beliefs, and feelings individuals have towards their spouse, their own marriage or marriage as an institution.

Family variables refer to any measurement of any aspect of a person's status with regard to relatives whether biological or adoptive, excluding marital variables as defined above. Thus family variables are measures of a person in reference to other members of their family.

Community variables refer to any measurement of a person's status in reference to the community. Community is defined in terms of five primary institutions of the community—job, residence, school, government, and religion.

These variables can have one of a number of roles in a given study. A central variable would be a focus of the study. A peripheral variable would be one that is measured and analyzed but only as a secondary concern. A covariate is a variable that is used to statistically match subjects or to provide statistical control of a variable thought to possibly confound the results of the study. An inclusion/exclusion variable is one used to define the sample. And a demographic variable is one used only for a description of the sample. Since most studies may have included more than a single family, marital, or community variable, the variables reviewed presently could have been used for any of the above capacities.

Studies versus Articles. An article is the term we use to refer to a published manuscript. However, some articles contain more than one study. Throughout this report we make the distinction between an article and a study.

Index of Emphasis. One goal of the present set of systematic reviews is to study the degree to which family, marital, and community variables are represented in each of the fields. There are a number of possible indices of this construct. The degree to which a particular field studies a class of variables can be measured by either the number of studies which have such a variable, or by the degree to which these variables are a central focus of the studies which include them. We have combined these two measures into an Index of Emphasis (IE) by multiplying the prevalence of studies by the proportion of variables in each class that are central. This number is then multiplied by 100 to result in an index that ranges from 0 for no emphasis (no inclusion whatsoever or no central variables) to 100 for total emphasis (every study had a variable and all variables were central):

IE = 100 * (proportion of included articles) * (proportion of central variables)

Quality of Research Methodology Index. When attempting to assess the quality of a research literature, it is difficult to determine an overall quality, due to a lack of available measurement strategies. To address this shortcoming, we have developed a 10-point scale of the quality of research methods to allow for comparisons of the quality of research between research in this review and others and between funded and unfunded research within this review (Lyons, Anderson, Larson, Penner, 1993). A study received one point for each of the following 10 characteristics, developed in part from Cook and Campbell (1979), if it were present:

Specification of gender and race of subjects (.5 points each)
Specification of sample frame
Specification of response rate
Use of prospective design
Use of multivariate statistics (0.5 points for univariate)
Absence of fishing/error rate threat
Sufficient statistical power
Absence of mono-method bias
Absence of ambiguity about direction of causal inference
Specification of reliability of at least one measure

If a study was purely descriptive it was given 0.5 points on fishing/error rate and statistical power ratings. These 10 characteristics, albeit somewhat lenient, were chosen based on experience with more than 10,000 articles reviewed. Further details on the definitions of these characteristics are available from the authors. Any empirical study, regardless of its research question or design can be rated on these characteristics. These characteristics were rated with a reliability of .96 for the present review.

In the present review, threats to validity were rated for studies with at least one central family, marital, or community variable. In addition, rating of threats were made for a set of randomly selected articles (see below) from each field.

Valence Definitions. The association of each of the identified variables with a given field's primary outcome was rated in terms of its valence—beneficial, neutral, harmful, mixed, or not assessed. This technique is consistent with the 'box score' strategy described by Glass, McGaw and Smith (1981). In order to maintain consistency so that each valence rating would have comparable meaning across studies, variables were rated in terms of the direction of their relationship with outcome measures of the field. Variable names are used to indicate the high end of the continuum on that variable. That is, for a variable called 'Socio-economic status,' a high score on that variable would indicate higher SES. Alternatively, for a variable called 'no family history of mental illness,' a high score would indicate no family history.

The association of these variables to field outcome assessments were then made such that beneficial was used when a high score on the variable was associated with a more positive outcome; neutral indicated no relationship, harmful indicated that a high score was associated with less positive outcome. Outcomes were unique to each field and were defined in terms of the primary focus of that field. Thus a variable named 'parental communication' would be rated as beneficial in the review of medicine or public health if it had a statistically significant relationship in which **higher levels of parental communication** was associated with **higher levels of health status**. It would be rated as neutral if there was no statistical association between these variables. It would be harmful when **higher levels of parental communication** was associated with **lower levels of health status**. The rating of not assessed is used to indicate that the authors did not describe the nature of the relationship between the family, marital or community variable and health, did not test this relationship statistically, or if the family, marital or community variable was a dependent measure. 'Not assessed' was also used to rate relationships that were judged not relevant to the primary field outcome.

Assessments of statistically significant interactions would fall under the category of 'mixed.' This category was used when a variable had a 'beneficial' association for one group and a 'harmful' association for a different group. Further, the valence of a particular variable was rated

48

based on multivariate associations if both univariate and multivariate analyses were reported.

Reliability of the Review. A central feature of systematic reviews is the reliability with which the review criteria are applied. For the present review step, training continued until reviewers had reliabilities of greater than 0.90 for each of the three components of the review. To insure against reliability decay, a random sample of 5 articles were re-reviewed each month and the reliability of the reviewers was re-assessed. The average reliability of the three components of the present review across all twenty fields was 0.95.

RESULTS

Prevalence of Research. Table 2 presents the prevalence of family, marital, and community research in eighteen of the twenty fields. Family research and family therapy research were excluded since 100% of the research in these fields includes the identified family and marital variables. Likewise, community variables were not reviewed within economics.

The fields with the greatest representation of family variables were Child Development, Clinical Psychology, and Sociology; each with more than one-third of their quantitative articles including a family variable. Political Science, Business, Law, and Education had the least representative with less than 15% of quantitative articles including a family variable.

Sex and Health Services both had more than one-third of their quantitative articles including marital variables. However, a number of fields had very few articles that included any marital measure whatsoever. Rehabilitation, Education, Political Science, Medicine, and Business had marital variables in less than 10% of quantitative articles.

A number of fields were found to have more than one-third of quantitative studies including community variables—Urban Planning had more than three-quarters, Sociology, Clinical Psychology, and Health Services also had high representation with more than one-half of quantitative studies including a community variable. Only two fields—Medicine and Geriatrics, had fewer than 20% of quantitative studies including a community variable.

Proportion of Central Variables. Table 3 presents the proportion of family, marital and community variables which were central to the article in which they were included. Compared to Table 2 which reports how often these variables were included in articles, these proportions indicate the degree to which family, marital, and community variables were emphasized in the articles where they were included.

Family variables were central more than two-thirds of the time that they were included in three fields—Law, Substance Abuse, and Sex. In Medicine, studied family variables were central less than one-third of the time.

TABLE 2. PREVALENCE OF FAMILY, MARITAL, AND COMMUNITY STUDIES ACROSS EIGHTEEN FIELDS

Field	Proportion of Empirical Studies		
	Family	Marital	Community
Education	.130	.020	.277
Business	.086	.052	.379
Child Development	.574	.106	.328
Clinical Psychology	.426	.285	.557
Communications	.173	.235	.359
Economics	.333	.323	.475
Geriatrics	.301	.281	.128
Health Services	.265	.369	.549
Law	.119	.153	.392
Medicine	.168	.047	.121
Political Science	.075	.021	.388
Psychiatry	.281	.159	.255
Public Health	.229	.159	.302
Rehabilitation	.230	.018	.317
Sex	.342	.456	.516
Sociology	.349	.240	.682
Substance Abuse	.326	.296	.452
Urban Planning	.176	.119	.766

TABLE 3. PROPORTION OF CENTRAL OF FAMILY, MARITAL, AND COMMUNITY STUDIES ACROSS EIGHTEEN FIELDS

Field	Proportion of Central Variables		
	Family	Marital	Community
Education	.347	.000	.303
Business	.448	.350	.540
Child Development	.457	.384	.188
Clinical Psychology	.452	.370	.170
Communications	.344	.507	.347
Economics	.678	.308	—
Geriatrics	.529	.288	.293
Health Services	.616	.632	.587
Law	.707	.638	.503
Medicine	.304	.035	.142
Political Science	.457	.250	.369
Psychiatry	.577	.238	.303
Public Health	.487	.341	.343
Rehabilitation	.579	.500	.571
Sex	.702	.489	.320
Sociology	.568	.605	.545
Substance Abuse	.748	.569	.532
Urban Planning	.544	.486	.624

Marital variables were central more than two-thirds of the time that they were included for Law and Health Services. On the other hand, Education had no central variables and Medicine had less than 10%.

Results for the centrality of community variables were consistent with the prevalence findings. Community variables were never central more than two-thirds of the time in any field. Not surprisingly, they were most often central in Urban Planning. Medicine, Clinical Psychology, and Child Development had the lowest proportion of central community variables each with less than 20%.

Index of Emphasis. Table 4 presents the Index of Emphasis which, as defined above, is the product of the proportions in Tables 2 and 3 multiplied by 100. For family variables, Child Development, Sex, Substance Abuse, and Sociology had the highest emphasis on these variables. Political Science, Business, Education, Medicine, and Communications had very little emphasis.

For research on marital variables, the overall emphasis was less than for family but Health Services and Sex had fairly high indices. Education and Medicine had no emphasis whatsoever; and, Political Science, Rehabilitation, and Business had very little.

In general, community variables were emphasized more than either family or marital variables. Urban Planning had the highest index score while

Sociology, Health Services, and Substance Abuse also demonstrated considerable emphasis. Medicine, Geriatrics, and Education had the three lowest levels of emphasis on community variables.

Proportion of Beneficial Variables. Table 5 presents the proportion of assessed variables that were found to have a beneficial association with the primary outcome in each field. If a variable was a dependent measure or if no statistical comparisons were made with the variable and a measure of outcome, then that variable was rated as 'not assessed.' Thus Table 5 is the proportion of assessed variables that were rated as beneficial (e.g., strong family associated with good outcome). This proportion gives an estimate of the relative 'potency' of families in research in each area.

For family research, the most consistent benefit was seen in Education, Medicine, Political Science, Child Development, and Public Health. The lowest levels of benefit (less than half of the assessed variables) was seen in the fields of Communications, Law, Health Services, Urban Planning, Sociology, and Geriatrics.

Among the marital variables studied, the most consistent benefit was reported in Urban Planning, Sex, and Clinical Psychology. Low levels of benefit were reported in Business, Psychiatry, Geriatrics, and Substance Abuse.

TABLE 4. INDEX OF EMPHASIS OF FAMILY/MARITAL/ COMMUNITY VARIABLES IN EACH OF EIGHTEEN FIELDS OF INQUIRY

Field	Index of Emphasis		
	Family	Marital	Community
Education	5	0	8
Business	4	2	20
Child Development	26	4	10
Clinical Psychology	19	11	10
Communications	6	12	12
Economics	23	10	—
Geriatrics	16	8	4
Health Services	16	23	32
Law	8	10	20
Medicine	5	0	2
Political Science	3	1	14
Psychiatry	16	4	8
Public Health	11	5	10
Rehabilitation	13	1	18
Sex	24	22	17
Sociology	20	15	37
Substance Abuse	24	17	24
Urban Planning	10	6	48

TABLE 5. PROPORTION OF BENEFICIAL VALENCES FOR CENTRAL OF FAMILY, MARITAL, AND COMMUNITY VARIABLES ACROSS EIGHTEEN FIELDS

Field	Proportion of Beneficial Central Variables		
	Family	Marital	Community
Education	.833	____*	.556
Business	.500	.333	.560
Child Development	.730	.526	.515
Clinical Psychology	.584	.571	.484
Communications	.333	.400	.500
Economics	.517	.454	
Geriatrics	.492	.357	.467
Health Services	.467	.541	.358
Law	.417	.529	.368
Medicine	.852	____*	.857
Political Science	.857	1.00**	.692
Psychiatry	.580	.333	.277
Public Health	.624	.475	.543
Rehabilitation	.590	.000**	.750
Sex	.512	.609	.585
Sociology	.441	.418	.375
Substance Abuse	.568	.361	.442
Urban Planning	.421	.750	.453

* no assessed central variables
** based on only one assessed central variable

TABLE 6. INDEX OF METHODOLOGICAL QUALITY: COMPARISON BETWEEN STUDIES WITH FAMILY/MARITAL/COMMUNITY VARIABLES AND RANDOMLY SELECTED STUDIES ACROSS THE TWENTY FIELDS OF INQUIRY

FIELD	Random Studies			Review Studies		
	MEAN	SD	RANGE	MEAN	SD	RANGE
1. Substance Abuse	5.27	1.39	3.0–8.5	5.10	1.44	1.0–8.5
2. Geriatrics	5.08	1.42	2.5–8.5	4.81	1.10	1.0–8.5
3. Family Therapy	4.91	1.12	2.0–8.5	—	—	—
4. Clinical Psychology	4.82	1.62	1.5–8.0	4.89	1.39	2.0–8.0
5. Public Health	4.80	1.24	2.0–7.5	4.92	1.24	2.0–7.5
6. Health Services	4.79	1.60	2.0–8.5	4.83	1.35	1.5–8.5
7. Psychiatry	4.78	1.20	1.5–7.5	4.66	1.47	1.0–8.0
8. Rehabilitation	4.69	1.24	2.0–7.5	4.88	1.21	2.0–7.5
9. Sex	4.66	1.22	2.5–8.5	4.41	1.31	1.5–8.5
10. Medicine	4.63	1.10	2.5–7.0	6.58*	0.90	5.5–8.5
11. Family Research	4.55	1.15	1.0–7.5	—	—	—
12. Business	4.55	1.31	1.0–7.0	4.83	1.26	2.0–7.5
13. Child Development	4.54	1.36	2.0–8.5	4.99*	1.32	1.0–8.5
14. Education	4.27	1.20	2.5–8.0	4.91*	1.70	2.0–8.5
15. Law	4.18	1.61	1.0–8.0	4.84*	1.55	2.0–9.0
16. Sociology	4.10	1.07	2.0–6.5	3.92	1.15	1.5–8.0
17. Communications	3.90	1.10	1.0–6.0	3.42*	1.42	1.0–6.5
18. Urban Planning	3.77	1.05	2.0–6.5	3.72	1.15	1.0–6.0
19. Economics	3.68	1.10	2.0–6.5	3.59	1.07	1.0–7.0
20. Political Science	3.59	1.28	2.0–7.0	3.47	1.18	1.0–7.0

Note: Family Therapy and Family Research estimates are based on all studies during the five year period therefore a comparison with randomly selected studies is not meaningful.
* different from the randomly selected studies p < .05

For community research, consistent benefit was reported in Medicine, Rehabilitation, and Political Science. Low levels of benefit were reported in Psychiatry, Health Services, Law, and Sociology.

Quality of Methodology. Table 6 presents a ranking of the twenty areas in terms of the quality of their methodology as described above using randomly selected articles from each field. Substance Abuse was the top rate field and Political Science was the lowest. The three lowest rated fields—Urban Planning, Economics, and Political Science, generally owed their rankings to the fact that studies failed to specify sample characteristics, did not report reliability of measures, and seldom used prospective designs. In general the fields that focused on health and mental health were higher rated than the other fields.

Comparison of the random study quality to the review articles reveals several interesting findings. In general quality was similar; however, for five fields the reviewed studies were of significantly different methodological quality compared to the randomly selected studies. In Medicine, Child Development, Education, and Law, the studies with a central family, marital, or community variable were of significantly higher methodological quality. In Communications, the review studies were of significantly lower methodological quality.

Federal Funding. Table 7 presents the proportion of articles including family, marital, or community variables that received at least partial support from the federal government through grants or contracts. The proportion of the randomly selected sample of articles is also included in the table.

In most cases, studies with family variables were more likely or equally likely to have been supported by federal monies than the random articles. Geriatrics had the largest difference with 41% of family articles having federal support compared to 24% of the random articles. Public Health, Clinical Psychology, Sex, and Medicine also had large differences. Among family research only Urban Planning and Sociology had notably lower proportion of federally supported research compared to the randomly selected articles.

The comparison of marital research to the random articles was similar to that of the family research except that Education and Rehabilitation had lower rates than the random articles, the opposite as that observed for family research.

In the fields of Business, Medicine, Clinical Psychology, Geriatrics, and Public Health research that included at least one community variable was more likely to be federally funded. The opposite was true for Education and Sociology.

Table 8 presents comparisons within each review of the quality of methodology for federally

TABLE 7. PROPORTION OF STUDIES RECEIVING FEDERAL FUNDING BY FIELD

	Family	Marital	Community	Random
Business	.14	.08	.19	.05
Child Development	.46	.51	.42	.41
Clinical Psychology	.62	.55	.57	.47
Communication	.16	.13	.21	.11
Economics	.52	.50	—	.38
Education	.32	.00	.17	.23
Geriatrics	.41	.45	.43	.24
Health Services	.50	.54	.52	.48
Family & Marriage	.18	.18	—	.19
Law	.41	.41	.45	.36
Medicine	.52	.61	.61	.34
Political Science	.33	.20	.27	.28
Psychiatry	.46	.42	.44	.42
Public Health	.45	.47	.44	.26
Rehabilitation	.26	.11	.26	.17
Sex	.18	.14	.14	.06
Sociology	.46	.52	.44	.57
Substance Abuse	.48	.43	.43	.42
Urban Planning	.08	.15	.11	.14

funded research versus research where no funding source was indicated. These comparisons were accomplished separately for family, marital, and community studies and for the randomly selected studies.

In four of the fields, a federal funding source was associated with increased quality as evidenced by the randomly selected articles. These fields were Clinical Psychology, Health Services, Medicine, and Sociology. Federal funding in the two family fields was also associated with higher methodological quality.

In addition to the Family/Marriage research field, federal funding was associated with higher methodological quality of family research in Health Services and Public Health and there was a trend towards high quality in Substance Abuse and Sociology. For marital research, federal funding was associated with high methodological quality in Family/Marriage, Health Services, and

TABLE 8. THE EFFECTS OF FEDERAL FUNDING ON THE QUALITY OF RESEARCH METHODOLOGY

Field	Family	Marital	Community	Random
Business	N.S.	N.S.	N.S.	N.S.
Child Development	N.S.	N.S.	N.S.	N.S.
Clinical Psychology	N.S.	N.S.	N.S.	2.03**
Communication	N.S.	N.S.	N.S.	N.S.
Economics	N.S.	N.S.	—	N.S.
Education	N.S.	—	N.S.	N.S.
Family Therapy	N.S.	N.S.	2.81***	—
Family Research	2.08**	2.74***	2.57**	—
Geriatrics	N.S.	N.S.	N.S.	N.S.
Health Services	2.22**	2.30**	2.71***	3.24***
Law	N.S.	N.S.	N.S.	N.S.
Medicine	N.S.	2.08*	N.S.	2.19**
Political Science	N.S.	—	N.S.	N.S.
Psychiatry	N.S.	N.S.	N.S.	N.S.
Public Health	2.09**	1.93*	N.S.	N.S.
Rehabilitation	N.S.	—	N.S.	N.S.
Sex	N.S.	N.S.	N.S.	N.S.
Sociology	1.95*	2.02**	2.34**	2.48**
Substance Abuse	1.68*	N.S.	N.S.	N.S.
Urban Planning	N.S.	N.S.	N.S.	N.S.

*p < .10
**p < .05
***p < .01

Sociology with a trend towards high quality in marital research in the Public Health Field. For community research, federal funding was associated with higher quality in Family Therapy, Family/Marriage Research, Health Services and Sociology.

BRIEF SUMMARIES OF THE INDIVIDUAL REVIEWS

The following are brief summaries of the findings from each field. Detailed analyses can be found in the accompanying detailed presentation of findings.

Business

The Business journals gave limited study to family and marital research, but more attention to community variables. The research in Business, on average, used adequate samples (median = 200), and studied more males than females (56% to 44%). The representation of minorities was slightly below national averages (African Americans were 8% of the samples, Hispanics were also 8%). The average age of subjects was 36.

Business studies failed to report the response rate 51% of the time, but when they did it was an adequate 73% average. Random sample frames were fairly common at 20%, but sample frames were not indicated in 50% of the studies. The best feature of the family, marital, and community research in the Business journals was that 58% of these articles reported some data on reliability. This rate was among the highest for all twenty fields.

Comparing the Business research in general, family research in Business had greater female representation (57% to 43%). Marital research had a similar gender proportion. Most troubling, in 85% of the studies including a family variable, the authors failed to indicate the racial/ethnic composition of their sample.

In terms of findings, there was little of note regarding family variables: few were assessed and no variable that was included in more than one study had a beneficial valence. For marital variables, being married was assessed more than once and had a beneficial valence. Spouse employed was assessed once and had a harmful valence.

Among community variables, job performance was consistently beneficial (5 of 5 times assessed). However, job tenure was reported beneficial 9 times, neutral six times, and harmful 3 times. Although higher income was not always beneficial

(6 of 11 times assessed), higher satisfaction with income always was (4 of 4 times assessed).

Child Development

This field had quite high inclusion of family variables, little attention to marital variables, and some attention to community variables. Sample sizes were smaller than other fields with a median of 112. Both genders were equally represented in the identified studies. The average age of the subjects was 9 years. The representation of African Americans was above the national average at 16%, but representation of Hispanics was low at 2%.

Random samples were rare and sampling frame was not indicated in two-thirds of the studies. Response rates were unreported in about two-thirds of the studies. Reliability was reported in more than three-quarters of the studies. Most of the research was cross-sectional.

For family and community research, the studies were consistent with those reported for all reviewed articles. Research that included marital variables, had a higher average age (14 years) and a greater representation of women (54% to 46%).

In terms of findings, parents' perceptions of child's behavior was seen as quite beneficial (12 beneficial, 1 mixed); family support was similar (14 beneficial, 1 neutral, 2 mixed), as was family relationship (15 beneficial, 3 neutral, 1 mixed). Family education/support programs were the most consistently beneficial (7 of 7 times assessed). No family disruption and no maternal depression were the next most consistently beneficial (5 of 5 times assessed). Maternal age was always neutral (4 of 4 times assessed) which indicates that this variable could well be irrelevant to child development outcomes.

No marital conflict was consistently beneficial although relatively unstudied (2 of 2 times assessed) as was spouse support (1 of 1 time assessed).

Socio-economic status was beneficial half the time (9 of 18, 8 neutral, and 1 mixed). Community stability was a beneficial community variable, but it was assessed only once.

Clinical Psychology

Clinical psychology had consistently high representations of all three classes of variables, although this field was not the highest on any of the measures of emphasis. The sample sizes for included articles were relatively small (median =

104). Females and males were equally represented and the average age of subjects was 31 years. Representation of minorities was near the national averages as samples were 17% African American and 6% Hispanic, although 54% of studies failed to indicate ethnicity/race composition of their samples.

Random samples were rare (8%), but authors generally indicated what sample frame was used (67%). Prospective studies were fairly common (44%) while retrospective studies were quite uncommon (3%).

Family research was quite comparable on the characteristics of all family, marital, and community articles. The only notable difference is that females were slightly over-represented (53% to 47%). This was also true for marital research (56% to 44%). However, in marital research Caucasians made up a larger proportion of the samples in general (80%) and African Americans and Hispanics were less well represented (11% and 2%, respectively). Community research was quite comparable to the overall characteristics and displayed no change in the sample demographics.

Few family variables were studied more than once. Six out of seven times, family education/support programs were reported to have beneficial effects (one neutral). Low levels of family stress was beneficial in 2 of 3 studies (1 neutral).

The absence of spousal aggression/violence was consistently rated as beneficial although it was only assessed twice. Marital status was neutral in each of the four studies where its association to mental health was assessed. The absence of mental illness in a spouse was beneficial in five studies and mixed in one other.

Work stability and rural residence were both consistently beneficial although seldom studied (2 of 2 and 1 of 1, respectively). Education level had quite mixed results.

Communication

This field had somewhat lower quality research and did not include many family or marital variables. Females were over-sampled in the family, marital, and community studies (57% to 43%), although this was not observed in the randomly selected studies. The average age was 29 years old. When noted, minorities were appropriately represented although only 4% were specifically identified as Hispanic. Unfortunately 85% of these studies failed to note ethnic/racial composition of the sample, suggesting that this field's performance on demographic representativeness may not be as favorable as the reported data suggests. In the randomly selected studies, 93% failed to report race/ethnicity.

Although random sample frames for the family studies were fairly frequent (27%), prospective studies were quite rare (5%). Most family research was based on cross-sectional or retrospective designs. Similar patterns of design were observed for marital and community studies.

Only two family variables were assessed among those that were included in more than one study. Both of these variables (number of children and positive feeling about abortion) were neutral. Marital satisfaction, although assessed only twice, was uniformly beneficial.

There was also relatively little attention to community variables. Educational status was assessed in 11 studies and was rated as beneficial six times, neutral three, and mixed twice. SES was rated as beneficial twice and mixed once.

Economics

This field is statistically quite sophisticated but otherwise methodologically weak. Family and marital variables were included in a fair proportion of studies. However, the specification of methodology and measurement was generally absent. In fact, not a single study (either included in the review or randomly selected) mentioned or referred to the reliability of any measurement used.

Most assessed family variables were neutral with the exception of lower number of children which was rated as beneficial in 7 of 8 instances. Younger parental age was beneficial once and neutral once. Larger extended family was neutral once and harmful once. The only marital variable used in more than one study was marital status. Being married was rated as beneficial 4 times, neutral 4 times, and harmful twice.

Education

Education research had a surprisingly low representation of family and marital variables. Also relative to many of the other fields, there was not a great deal of attention to community variables (despite the fact that educational outcome was considered a community variable in the present review). The methodological quality was somewhat low in general and not particularly improved within the family, marital, and community research.

Education research included in the present review tended to have large samples (median = 430) and females were included more than males (60% to 40%). The average age was 13. Although 58% of studies failed to indicate the racial/ethnic composition of samples, when indicated, minorities were well represented with 21% African American and 12% Hispanic.

Random sample frames were used in 17% of studies and prospective designs were used in 38% of studies. Reliability was reported in 44% of the research included in the review.

When family variables were studied they had nearly uniformly positive association with educational outcomes. In 15 of 19 comparisons, the family variables were rated as beneficial.

Geriatrics

Only the top two geriatrics journals were reviewed as the third journal had recently divided itself into multiple journals (appearing in a single issue). Therefore, any observed changes over the 1986 to 1990 time frame of the review would have been difficult to interpret and aggregate data from across that time period would not be useful.

In general the quality of methods used in geriatrics was quite good. There was considerable inclusion of family and marital variables, although the field did not include as many community variables as compared to some of the other fields.

Consistent with demographic trends among the elderly, subjects in the reviewed articles were predominantly women (64% to 36%). The average age was 67. Minorities were adequately represented at 12% African American and 5% Hispanic.

Random sample frames were fairly common (20%), and 80% of studies indicated what sample frame was used. Over half of the studies were cross-sectional (53%), although a significant portion were prospective (28%).

The separate family, marital, and community studies all mirrored these sample and design characteristics closely.

Among the family research studies, the majority of harmful findings involved the effects of burden on family members of caring for a medically ill older adult. Being a caregiver was rated as harmful in 10 out of 20 assessed variables. This variable was rated as mixed five times and was found to be beneficial only once. Consistent with other fields, educational and supportive interventions were found to be consistently beneficial (11 of 16 times assessed).

Among marital variables, marital status was generally neutral (15 of 27 times), although it was rated as beneficial in seven studies. As with family caregiver, a spousal caregiver was consistently associated with harmful effects (on the caregiver) in 3 of 8 studies with 3 more studies rated as mixed.

Most community variables were predominantly neutral. Although income was beneficial in 12 instances out of 27, it was neutral in 14. Likewise educational level was beneficial in 11 instances, neutral in 11, harmful in 2 and mixed in 2. Residential arrangement (living in the community vs in an institution) was rated as the most consistently beneficial (7 out of 9 with 1 neutral and 1 mixed).

Health Services

Health services research was generally of fairly high quality and included considerable representation of family, marital, and community variables. The samples were generally quite large (median = 1,688). Females were more highly represented than males (54% to 46%). The average age was 51 years old. Nearly three-quarters of the studies (73%) failed to present the ethnic/racial composition of their sample. However when indicated, the percentages of African Americans (13%) were consistent with national averages although the number of Hispanics (4%) was an under-representation.

Random sample frames were used in nearly one third of studies. Prospective designs were used in one-fifth of studies. Only 18% of studies made any reference to the reliability of measures.

Separate analyses of research that used either family, marital, or community variables were comparable in the above characteristics, although the average age of the subjects of the family research was a bit lower at 46 years and Hispanics were almost completely unrepresented (1%).

Among the findings of the family research, parental education was always assessed as beneficial (3 of 3). Parental influence was also uniformly beneficial (2 of 2).

Being married was associated with a better health care outcome in 18 of 33 studies. This variable was neutral in 12 cases, harmful in 1 and mixed in 2.

For community variables, the most commonly studied variables were income (beneficial in 15, neutral in 17 and harmful in 6) and education (beneficial in 12, neutral in 15 and harmful in 2).

Living in a rural versus urban setting did not appear to effect health outcomes (beneficial 2, neutral 11, harmful 3). Receiving public assistance was beneficial in 8 of 18 studies (neutral in 7, harmful in 2, and mixed in 1).

Law

This review was somewhat complicated by the fact that very little empirical research appears in law journals. The vast majority of commonly cited journals in this field are review journals established by law schools. Thus the journals used presently ranged from a commonly cited journal to one that is not often cited relative to other journals in the field.

Within the quantitative studies included in the present review, the samples were generally large (median = 293) and predominantly male (65% to 35%). The average age was 31. Although the racial/ethnic composition was missing in 63% of the studies, the representation of African Americans was quite high (31%). Hispanics were under-represented (2%) compared to national averages.

Random samples were used in 13% of the family, 11% of the marital, and 15% of the community studies. Prospective designs were used in 16%, 15%, and 17% of the family, marital, and community studies, respectively.

Of the family variables that appeared in more than one study, the following were uniformly beneficial (although each was assessed only once): no abuse, family stability, no running away, parental supervision. Living with family and more parental influence were harmful in the three studies where they were assessed. No spouse abuse was beneficial in the one study where it was assessed, while being married was beneficial in 3 studies, neutral in 2 and mixed in one.

For the community studies, higher levels of income, SES, or education were generally neutral in their associations with legal outcomes. Community variables were frequently not assessed in terms of their associations with legal outcomes.

Medicine

Given the weekly publication of the top two journals in Medicine, a random one third sample of the published research from 1986 through 1990 was selected. Review of these studies revealed some attention to family and community variables and little attention to marital variables.

The sample sizes of review articles were generally large (median = 572) and predominantly female (61% to 39%). This gender distribution is in dramatic comparison to the randomly selected general articles in Medicine which had 58% male samples. This difference is predominantly explained by the presence of pregnancy and child birth research in medicine. Thus, the overall under-representation of women in medical research is not observed within family, marital, and community research in medicine. Nearly two-thirds of studies (63%) failed to indicate racial/ethnic composition.

In terms of findings for family research, no prenatal exposure to drugs was uniformly beneficial (5 of 5 times assessed). No general family history of medical illness was beneficial in 4 studies and mixed in one. No disease when pregnant was beneficial in five studies and neutral in one. Family involvement was beneficial the two times it was assessed. There were no assessed marital variables.

For community research, income was beneficial in two studies and vocational training was beneficial the one time it was assessed. Living in a rural location was harmful in the one instance where it was assessed.

Political Science

This field had the overall lowest quality of research. This was partially due to its reliance on cross-sectional and retrospective designs and the general failure to report reliability of measures. Sample sizes were generally quite large (median = 1,241) and gender distribution was relatively even (52% male: 48% female). The average age of subjects was 48 years old. Very few studies reported the racial ethnic composition of samples (8%).

While community research was common, family and marital research were rare in this field. Only three family variables were included in more than one study and each was assessed only once—all were beneficial. These variables were high paternal occupational status, fewer number of abortions, and more positive feelings about abortion.

Higher education (9 of 11), higher occupational status (3 of 3) and higher income (9 of 14) were often beneficial. Higher SES was beneficial in 3 studies and harmful in 3 other studies. Income equality was uniformly beneficial (4 of 4 studies). Religiosity was beneficial in the two instances it was assessed.

ST. OLAF COLLEGE LIBRARIES

Psychiatry

Like medicine, the volume of quantitative articles required the use of a random sample of articles for the review. A 50% sample from the top three journals was used. Psychiatry had a fairly good representation of family and community variables and was average on the inclusion of marital variables.

In the articles included in the review, samples sizes were relatively small (median = 110). The relative proportion of male and female subjects was fairly even (51% female to 49% male). Two-thirds of the studies failed to describe the racial/ethnic composition of their samples; however, in those that did, African Americans made up 11% and Hispanics 3% of subjects. Family and marital research were similar to these overall characteristics. Community research had a somewhat greater representation of men (53%).

Random selection was quite rare (3%) and sample frames were not indicated in 33% of studies. Prospective designs were fairly common (28%). Reliability was reported for at least one measure in 37% of studies.

Among the findings, family history variables were the most commonly studied family variables. In 29 of 36 assessments, no family history of psychiatric illness was rated as beneficial (neutral in the remaining 7). In 8 of 13 assessments no family history of substance abuse was rated as beneficial (5 neutral). A number of other family variables were uniformly beneficial: maternal emotion (4 of 4), no childhood neglect (3 of 3), family education (2 of 2), adjustment to death (2 of 2). Number of children was neutral in 5 of 6 assessments. Marital status was neutral in 8 of 11 assessments. No history of prior marriages was beneficial in the one study that assessed this variable.

Income (3 of 3), education (9 of 11), employment status (5 of 5) and SES (4 of 6) were generally neutral—unrelated to mental health outcomes. Not being homeless and being in a vocational program were both beneficial in the individual studies that assessed these variables.

Public Health

Public health research which included family, marital, or community variables generally involved large samples (median = 1,104) and had proportionally more females than males (62% female, 38% male). Family research had a particularly high representation of women (72%). African Americans were represented as 21% of the samples on average and Hispanics were 10% of the samples. Other or unspecified nonwhites made up an additional 11% of samples.

Random samples were fairly common (26%) although one quarter of the studies failed to indicate the sample frame used. Prospective designs were used in 20% of the studies. Reliability was presented for at least one measure in 17% of studies.

In the family research findings, breast feeding was uniformly beneficial (5 of 5) as were the following other family variables: no family member smoking (4 of 4), longer birth interval (2 of 2), prenatal care (2 of 2), no family disruption (2 of 2), fewer siblings (2 of 2), pregnancy (2 of 2), planned pregnancy (2 of 2), not being a parent as a teen (2 of 2), educational program on pregnancy (2 of 2).

Being married was beneficial in 21 instances, neutral in 17, harmful in 7 and mixed in 1. Living with a spouse was neutral in the 3 instances it was assessed. Spousal influence was beneficial once and harmful once.

Not being homeless was uniformly beneficial (5 of 5). Income was beneficial 28 times, neutral 12 times, harmful 9 times, and mixed 3 times. Educational level was beneficial 34 times, neutral 20 times, harmful 4 times. Not on public assistance was beneficial twice and harmful three times. Job tenure was beneficial in the one study where it was assessed.

Rehabilitation

Rehabilitation appears overall to be somewhat more like education than like child development, although this field clearly falls between the two in its inclusion of family and marital variables. In general among the family, marital, or community articles, samples were small (median = 102) and males predominated (67% male to 33% female). Two-thirds of the studies failed to describe the racial/ethnic composition of their samples. For those studies that did, African Americans were 19% and Hispanics were 6% of the subjects. These basic demographics applied to the family, marital, and community studies separately as well.

Random sampling was fairly uncommon (12%) as were prospective designs (17%). The majority of research was cross-sectional (74%). About one-third of the studies (35%) reported the reliability of any measure.

A number of family variables were uniformly beneficial: maternal education (3 of 3), parental estimate of child's ability (2 of 2), no family conflict (2 of 2), family support (1 of 1), family stability (1 of 1). Marital variables were essentially unstudied—marital status was neutral in the one study in which it was assessed.

Vocational programs were uniformly beneficial (7 of 7) as was income (2 of 2), educational level (2 of 2), and living in the community (1 of 1). Rural residence was harmful in one study and mixed in another.

Sex

Perhaps not surprisingly, Sex research had the highest representation of marital variables. Family and community variables were also fairly well represented overall.

The median sample size was 132 with fairly equal representation of men (51%) and women (49%). The average age of subjects was 32.5 years. Nearly two-thirds of the samples failed to provide information on the racial/ethnic composition of samples. African Americans (8%) and Hispanics (3%) appear to be somewhat under-represented compared to national averages.

Random samples were rare (6%) and prospective designs were fairly uncommon (17%). Most research involved no or an unspecified sample frame (74%) and a cross-sectional design (70%). Reliability was reported on at least one variable in 36% of studies.

Sociology

Sociology generally used large samples (median = 1,613) and had a higher proportion of men (60%) than women (40%). The average age of subjects in the family, marital, or community studies was 30 years. Race/ethnicity was missing in 71% of the studies. In the remaining 29%, African Americans made up 16% of the sample and Hispanics 5%. Unspecified 'nonwhite' made up 28% of the reported samples.

Random samples were fairly common (24%) although 56% of studies failed to indicate a sample frame. Only 2% of studies were prospective. Reliability of any measure was reported in only 15% of studies.

Among the findings for family research, an intact home was beneficial in 9 of 11 instances (2 neutral). A number of family variables were uniformly beneficial: positive family relationship (6 of 6), longer birth interval (3 of 3), no family conflict (3 of 3), no family disruption (2 of 2), small-

er family size (2 of 2), no abuse in family (2 of 2), no parental criminal history (2 of 2).

A larger variety of marital variables were assessed in Sociology than in most of the other fields. Marital status was beneficial in 14 of 27 instances. A number of marital variables were uniformly beneficial: spouse's income (4 of 4), spouse's educational level (3 of 3), spouse's occupational level (2 of 2), living with spouse (2 of 2), no marital problems (1 of 1), spouse's religion (1 of 1), positive attitude toward marriage (1 of 1).

Many community variables were assessed. Income was beneficial in 40 of 60 assessments. Educational level was beneficial in 35 of 55. SES was beneficial in 10 of 22. Living in a rural location was beneficial 10 times and harmful 11 times. Some community variables were uniformly beneficial: educational aspiration (4 of 4), positive perception of employment (1 of 1). Number of women in the workforce was beneficial 5 of 6 times and harmful once.

Substance Abuse

This field had the highest quality of methodology rating and was among the highest in its representation of family, marital, and community research. Sample sizes were midrange (median = 205) and predominantly male (62% male, 38% female). The average age was 31 years. Almost half the studies report race/ethnicity. African Americans (15%) and Hispanics (8%) were well-represented. An additional average of 16% of subjects were an unspecified 'nonwhite' ethnicity.

Random samples were used in 13% of studies reviewed. Prospective designs were used in about one-third (34%). Reliability on at least one measure was reported in 43% of studies.

Far and away the most commonly assessed family variable was family history of substance abuse problems. In 71 instances no family history of substance abuse was found to be beneficial, 23 were neutral, 1 was harmful, and 2 were mixed. Few family variables were uniformly beneficial, indicating a complex literature in terms of the role of the family. Family independence was beneficial in the 3 instances it was assessed.

Marital variables were also somewhat inconsistent. Marital status was neutral in 25 of 38 assessments. Spouse not using alcohol was beneficial in 5 instances, neutral in 1 and mixed in 1 other. Spouse not smoking was beneficial in 3 and neutral in 3. In the one study that assessed spouse influences it was found to be beneficial.

The various community measures related to SES were generally neutral. Income was neutral in 10 of 19 assessments, educational level was neutral in 20 of 32, SES was neutral in 8 of 12. Thus, substance abuse problems do not appear to be related to SES and proxies. No school problems was uniformly beneficial (6 of 6). Religiosity was beneficial in 6 of 9 assessments (3 neutral).

Urban Planning

Urban planning had relatively low quality of methods. However, this field had the greatest inclusion of community variables. Family and marital variables were fairly well represented compared to the other fields. Sample sizes were midrange (n = 338) and predominantly male (64% male to 36% female). Age of subjects was not reported in 93% of studies and race/ethnicity was not reported in 87%. The few studies that did report race had substantial minority representation: 30% African American, 8% Hispanic, 32% unspecified 'nonwhite.'

Sample frames were occasionally random (13%). However only 1% of studies utilized prospective designs. The majority of studies used retrospective designs (80%). Reliability of any measure was reported in just 5% of reviewed studies.

MEASUREMENT IN MARITAL AND FAMILY RESEARCH

It is clear from the review of the use of family and marital variables in the above 18 fields that there is not a widespread dispersion of family and marital measures into other fields. In order to facilitate such a technology transfer, we have inventoried each of the measures used from 1986 to 1990 in the Family Research journals and the Family Therapy journals.

These compilations can be found in the reference material that accompanies this summary. Review of these tables of measures reveals that both fields, and particularly Family Research, frequently utilize idiosyncratic measurements that are designed specifically for the study at hand and seldom used again, except by the same investigators. There are notable exceptions to this practice: in Family Therapy, the Family Environment Scale (FES), the Family Adaptability and Cohesion Scales (FACES-II), and the Family Assessment Device (FAD). On the positive side, relia-

bility of measures was very often studied in both Family Research and Family Therapy.

SUMMARY

The preceding was a brief review of a large body of research spanning 20 different fields of inquiry. To summarize this research in a brief yet meaningful way represents a significant challenge. To devise recommendations for these data poses an even greater challenge.

First, it appears that family, marital, and community research has not broadly permeated most of the fields studied. While notable exceptions exist, a surprising neglect of these variables can be found in a number of fields. Education and Rehabilitation are notable examples. Both of these fields appear to generally view the educational process as one that occurs between the student and the teacher with little influence coming from the outside world of family and community. One wonders whether progress in these fields may be somewhat impeded by such a narrow definition of scope.

There was a surprising lack of information provided about subject demographic characteristics in general and race/ethnicity, specifically. In the majority of fields, less than one-half of the studies specified the racial composition of their samples. While, when indicated, the samples generally appeared to be representative of the cultural variation observed in the United States, concern regarding the overall representativeness is generated by the absence of information in the majority of studies.

Generally women were more commonly studied in family and marital research than men. This often occurred despite the fields' general over-sampling of men as demonstrated in the randomly selected articles. One reason for this phenomenon was that pregnancy was a commonly studied family variable. However, this does not appear to fully account for the demographic difference. Further investigation of the existing database is necessary to identify other factors that account for the sampling disparities between family and marital research specifically within the various fields.

Sometimes federal funding was associated with higher methodological quality and sometimes it was not. The Index of Methodological Quality is an indicator developed for this project and as such has not been widely studied. It is possible that the absence of differences is due in part to the instrument. However, the methodological standards enumerated in the index are not particularly controversial and represent rather minimal standards for quality. Thus the interpretation that federal funding is not invariably related to increased research quality is, at minimum, tenable. One caveat to this conclusion may be that federal funding may be used to stimulate research in under-studied areas or in complex areas in which good research methods are harder to apply. Unfortunately, this would not appear to be a useful explanation of why federally funded research failed to specify sample demographics or sample frames.

The policy implications of these comparisons are, at least, two-fold. In cases where federal funding is not associated with increased methodological quality, policy interventions might be directed at the review and funding process. Thus, in areas where funding is not associated with an improvement in quality, a call for improved oversight is reasonable. In areas where funding is associated with an increase in quality, a call for increased funding is more readily defensible.

There are a number of findings, similar across fields, that are worthy of note. It appears that the strength of family relationships as measured by a host of constructs including communication, influence, supervision, etc. is a potent variable in the health and well-being of persons living in the United States.

Measure of socio-economic status and proxies of this construct appear to have quite variable effects across fields. Unlike family relationship variables they are seldom uniformly beneficial in any fields. The idea that having more money or resources might sometimes be harmful may be counter-intuitive; however, results of this review suggest that circumstances exist where this is likely to be the case.

RECOMMENDATIONS

A number of recommendations can be made based on the findings of these systematic reviews.

First, the review of nearly 8000 articles on family, marital and community research has generated a significant database that can be used to pursue questions within or across fields. Some mechanism is necessary whereby this database can become accessible to scholars interested in pursuing lines of research addressed in the present review. Updating and expanding this database may also prove useful.

Second, the findings regarding the association of federal funding to research quality are quite provocative. Although in some cases receipt of federal funding may be associated with improved methodology, this was not uniformly the case. This suggests that more research dollars may not always translate into better research. With regards to family research per se, it does appear that research in that field is improved by federal funding. Particularly in areas that do not show methodological quality improvement with federal funding, guidelines regarding publication of federally funded research findings may be useful to address some of these methodological shortcomings. For example, the National Institute of Health requires specification of racial composition in proposed research. Such a guideline could be extended to research published from funded projects.

Third, dissemination of the results of these reviews to the fields studied is also highly recommended. This may be one mechanism for stimulating further study of these issues.

Fourth, the further development of measures useful to family, marital, and community researchers should be a priority. Most studies used simple measures, did not study or report their reliability or validity, and used mono-methods. The reviews of measures used in marital and family research and family therapy may prove useful to researchers in other fields. Family research appears to infrequently utilize common measurements. For the field to advance, researchers will need, at some point, to settle on common instrumentation so that findings across studies can be interpretable.

Fifth, a number of fields used large national databases as their primary sources. For example, in Economics, the majority of family and marital studies used the Michigan Panel Study of Income Dynamics. To stimulate these fields to engage in improved family, marital and community research, it would be most efficient to work to improve the measurement of relevant variables in these large national databases.

REFERENCES

Bareta, J. C., Larson, D. B., Lyons, J. S., & Zorc, J. (1990). A comparison of a MEDLARS and systematic review of the consultation-liaison literature. *American Journal of Psychiatry, 147,* 1040-1042.

Cook, T., & Campbell, D. T. (1979). *Quasi-experimentation. Design & analysis issues for field setting.* New York: Houghton, Mifflin.

Dagg, P. (1991). Psychological sequelae of abortion. *American Journal of Psychiatry, 148,* 578-585.

Glass, G. V., McGaw, B., & Smith, J. L. (1981). *Meta-analysis in social research*. Beverly Hills, CA: Sage.

Kazdin, A. E., Bass, D., Siegel, T., & Thomas, C. (1989). Cognitive-behavioral therapy and relationship therapy in treatment of children referred for antisocial behavior. *Journal of Consulting and Clinical Psychology, 57*, 522-535.

Larson, D. B., Lyons, J. S., Hohmann, A. A., Beardsley, R. S., Huckeba, W., Rabins, P. V., & Lebowitz, D. B. (1989). A systematic review of nursing home research in three psychiatric journals: 1966-1985. *International Journal of Geriatric Psychiatry, 4*, 129-134.

Larson, D. B., Kessler, L. C., Burns, B. J., et al. (1987). A research development workshop to stimulate outcome research in consultation-liaison psychiatry. *Hospital and Community Psychiatry, 38*, 1106-1109.

Larson, D. B., Sherrill, K. A., Lyons, J. S., Craigie, F. C., Thielman, S. B., Greenwold, M. A., & Larson, S. S. (1990). Associations between dimensions of religious commitment and mental health reported in the *American Journal of Psychiatry* and *Archives of General Psychiatry:* 1978-1989. *American Journal of Psychiatry, 149*, 557-559.

Lyons, J. S., Larson, D. B., Bareta, J. C., Liu, I., Anderson, R. L., & Sparks, C. H. (1990). A systematic analysis of the quantity of AIDS publications and the quality of research methods in three general medical journals. *Evaluation & Program Planning, 13*, 73-77.

Lyons, J. S., Anderson, R. L., & Larson, D. B. (1992). *A reliable index for assessing the methodological quality of a research literature*. Unpublished manuscript.

Lyons, J. S., Anderson, R. L., Larson, D. B., & Penner, J. (1992). Of parents and pocket-books: A systematic review of family, marital, and community variables in juvenile criminal justice research. Department of Justice.

Ney, P. G., & Wickett, A. R. (1989). Mental health and abortion: Review and analysis. *Psychiatric Journal of Ottawa, 14*, 506-516.

RON HASKINS, PH.D.
Welfare Counsel
Ways and Means Committee
U.S. House of Representatives

Research and the Political Process

I have bad news and good news. The bad news is that it is shocking how little I have to say that is relevant to the themes of this conference, but the good news is, I can barely talk, so I'm not going to be here long.

I am always happy to talk about research and policy, primarily because it is impossible to say anything very intelligible about what actually determines policy. So no matter what I say, none of you can prove me wrong. Unlike the other people in this room, I am a recovering social scientist. I came to Washington on a one-year AAAS fellowship determined to study the impact of social science research on policy formulation, and go back to the University of North Carolina to write the definitive book on the subject. That was in 1985.

That I am still here indicates the sad truth: the more I participate in the policy process, the less I understand about the impact of research on policy. But here is one thing I do understand: systematic reviews are interesting, but they suffer from the same flaw as traditional reviews and meta analyses: the review starts with a question. The kind of reviews we do on the Hill are much more efficient. We always start with the answer. Members of Congress decide in advance what the best policy is, usually on the basis of ideology. Now we can divide all the studies into two stacks, one stack of the good ones, and the other stack of the bad ones. Then they hire guys like me to show why the stack of good ones are pristine research and the bad ones are terribly flawed and need to be trashed. Indeed, that is why they send me to conferences like this, so I can get the individual goods on you.

The conclusion that this leads me to is that in politics, research is used like a weapon. So the way social scientists can have an impact is to achieve consensus. This way, it will be much more difficult for charlatans like me to foil you with our ideology.

In the field of intervention, the field I am most familiar with, the best way to achieve consensus is with experiment and random assignment. Experiments are hard for demographers, so the true path to consensus for demographers and perhaps other health researchers is replication. Thus, I think you should spend time here talking about how to achieve consensus based on replication. You're the experts on this, of course, but I would say there are at least two keys here, and I was very pleased to notice that both of them had been mentioned this morning.

The first is sampling. There has been a lot of talk here about sampling already, and I really don't have anything to add, except that if you don't get it right, you sow confusion and reap irrelevance. The second determinant is measures. I used to struggle with this sort of thing back when I was doing research as a developmental psychologist, but I always wound up with a headache, and I'm not sure I can do any better now. I learned as a graduate student that a good measure is one that is reliable and valid. Great. So where do you find such measures?

Now let me add, the three types of measures I think we most need to know about — and here I'm going to second Nick Zill — are parenting, peer influences and community organizations, especially churches. Families make a huge difference on all sorts of variables, including health. There has been too little discussion of that in this conference. There is research that goes back decades showing that families can have dramatic impacts even in the midst of the worst possible environmental conditions. I heard someone talking before the meeting started about the article in *Scientific American* recently about Asian families living in the deepest, darkest ghettos. They send their kids to school and they wind up being valedictorians. When they start, they cannot even speak English, they have been out of Vietnam for three years, spent two years in what amounts to a kind of concentration camp. Then they come to America and live in Dallas, Seattle, Fort Worth. Ten years later their kids are valedictorians. So researchers go and look at these families to see how they can produce such miracles. Here is what they find. After dinner, the family — the parents often don't speak English — clears the table, they put all the kids at the table and they stand there and encourage them to study. The older kids supervise the younger kids. All this is done through the context of family. The kids go to exactly the same schools as typical residents of inner cities, and yet they wind up going to great universities on scholarships. So families can overcome probably not all, but some dramatic difficulties.

Clearly, then, we need to have measures of family processes, exactly the thing that is most lacking in these surveys. Of those processes, I think there are several specific dimensions that we need to know how to measure. The first one is discipline. The second is absence of physical punishment. There is a huge amount of literature on this issue, and it shows that use of physical punishment has negative outcomes. The third is talk and discussion — amount of talk when kids are babies, but as they grow older, contingent talk, discussions, and adult expansions. Psycholinguists have nice ways to measure these types of language. A fourth dimension is parental warmth, which is shown over and over again to be quite critical to child development.

You can figure out how to operationalize these, and then get all your colleagues to agree that you have done it and relay to us your new measures. Then when you finish, you can proceed to figure out good measures for peer group influ-

ences and the developmental impact of community organizations. My IQ is way too low to say anything very constructive about peer influences, but I have one little thing to say about religion.

I think religion, like gangs, gives kids something to believe in. Recall that Congress doesn't need good literature reviews, because they already know the answer. Their ideology told them. We want kids to be the same way. They know it is wrong to be violent, to drink, to use drugs, to fornicate, because they carry a set of values that defines these things as wrong, period.

Now, some of you may be saying, great ideas, but try to get three questions that capture these constructs in a national survey of 5,000 people. Felicia LeClere is probably getting ready to throw me out of the room right now. You recall yesterday she made a comment about complexity making survey items too difficult to score. I assume you demographers have a sense of proportion. You know what can be reasonably accomplished in a national survey. Even so, consider these two points.

First, don't give up trying to find good measures of complex constructs that don't take two hours to administer and even more to score. The Caldwell-Bradley HOME measurement is a good example of what I have in mind. It is fairly short, and yet gives you a fairly good idea about what happens in a family. It is not perfect, but it is something that can be used in a national survey. I know other people have used it in national surveys, so it is possible to get at least some measurement of complex constructs in national surveys.

Second, there must be a way to coordinate demographic survey work with laboratory and large-scale experiments. That is why the public has put so much money for research in Health and Human Services (HHS). They know there is no rivalry among its various divisions, offices and branches, and that the coordination of research is a routine practice at HHS.

Finally, let me add something that at first seems to undermine everything I've said to this point. I know that the single most important characteristic about social science research and its connection with policy is this: simplicity. Einstein said, seek simplicity and distrust it. I say, seek simplicity and if you don't find it, seek some more. When you talk to policy makers, there are two issues that you must deal with. I'm going to call this a personality dimension. These are people who don't want complexity, don't like complexity. Yet they must deal with complexity all the time. Speaking of time, they don't have very much of it, so they're not going to read anything you write. They will simply tune it out. They will not allow you to make their lives more complex. The message must be simple.

Second, what we have in the United States Congress is a fairly good representation of the population on almost any characteristic you choose to name, including intelligence, but with the bottom of the distribution lopped off. So you're dealing with a tremendous range of thinking and commitment and so forth. Members of Congress are not going to be moved by systematic reviews. There are not more than one or two politicians in all of Congress who will ever read one of these things. So you will be at the mercy of staff. And if that doesn't scare you, staff means

guys like me who can put a spin on your message in a flash. So I absolutely promise you, simplicity of message is the key.

In summary, policy in fact depends on consensus among researchers. Without consensus, you will be undermined, in some cases by each other. Second, systematic reviews are good to the extent that they can convince scientists that consistency has been found across studies. That is, that replication is a fact and that it can lay the groundwork for consensus. Third, in addition to persuasive reviews, consensus can be achieved by more attention to samples and measures, and people should be spending money to do that.

Above all, finally, when you are communicating with policy makers, simplicity is a must. That is why I was the ideal person to make this presentation.

Kristin Moore, Ph.D.
Executive Director
Child Trends, Inc.

Family Strengths and Youth Behavior Problems,

Analyses of Three National Survey Databases

(Prepared under DHHS Contract HHS-100-92-0015 Delivery Order 02)

The news we get about American families is almost invariably bad. Whether it is a new statistical report or a story about a particular family, the news is worried at best, and often simply negative.

However, not all the news really is bad. When parents are asked about their own families and their relationships with their own children, their responses are generally very positive. For example, while parents report stress about time and about money, they nevertheless indicate strong feelings about their children and substantial involvement in their lives. Moreover, even many children growing up under adverse conditions have been found to be highly resilient. Similarly, a literature has developed that focuses on successful families and strong families.

This literature on family strengths has identified a set of characteristics that distinguish strong families. These constructs include communication among family members, the encouragement of the individuals in the family, a religious or spiritual orientation, social connectedness with community, neighbors and relatives, the ability to adapt to changing circumstances, expressing appreciation for other family members, clear roles within the family, and time together doing activities as a family or as groups within the family.

Researchers find considerable consensus across varied cultural groups regarding the characteristics of successful families. Indeed, it makes considerable intuitive sense that families who communicate, adapt, spend time together and express appreciation for one another would be stronger. Presumably adults in such families are happier or more satisfied, and similarly, the assumption has been widespread that children raised in families that have one or especially several family strengths would be happier and more successful themselves.

However, for a variety of reasons, the empirical case has been weak. In particular, our capacity to describe problems exceeds our capacity to understand the factors that explain normal or successful development, or to develop public or private interventions to enhance positive outcomes. Our limited understanding is attributable in part to the inadequacy of current data, both the kinds of family measures available and the samples themselves.

A preponderance of the studies about children and families are based on small and/or non-representative samples. For example, researchers studying the effects of day dare and maternal employment have tended to rely on white middle class samples drawn from child care centers, often high-quality, university-based programs. Studies that focus on average day care and studies of day care in low income and minority group samples, with a few recent exceptions, are rare. Similarly, some researchers studying the effects of divorce (e.g., Wallerstein & Kelly, 1980) have focussed on highly selective samples, such as families seeking clinical help. While studies based on delimited samples can be heuristic, they are too often used by researchers and policymakers to generalize to the larger population, where results derived from such sub-groups can be misleading.

Another shortcoming of available research is that studies tend to derive from a particular disciplinary perspective and researchers therefore focus on only a range of predictor variables. For example, researchers may focus on socioeconomic status to predict children's achievement, ignoring both the roles of neighborhood and community context and the role of family socialization practices. Other researchers may focus solely on family interaction patterns, paying little heed to the social context in which families develop these patterns. To inform our understanding of the factors that explain the trends occurring in children's lives in recent years, we need studies that examine, for example, both family dynamics and "policy" variables in the same models. Such multi-layered analyses would allow us to assess each set of influences, such as the family, the community, and peers net of the other factors as well as in interaction with them.

There is also a real need for prospective studies. Much of what we know about the factors associated with children's well-being is cross sectional in nature. That is, we are merely able to ascertain that a given characteristic is *correlated* with a particular child outcome. Longitudinal data that permit researchers to examine prospectively the factors and processes that *predict* to child outcomes are far too infrequent.

Differences in families within income, family structure and race/ethnicity groups often go unexplored. For example, studies of whites tend to be conducted among white middle class families, while studies of blacks tend to be conducted among low income and underclass families. Alternatively, families of varied types may be examined together, so that the processes important in single parent families, for example, cannot be distinguished from those that characterize two-parent families.

Contemporary research on families and children also tends to take a negative perspective. Studies tend to focus on family pathologies and problems, particularly among adolescents. Studies of normal development and positive family functioning constitute just a minority of the available literature.

THE CURRENT RESEARCH

The analyses conducted for this project address a portion of these concerns in that they focus on positive family characteristics; specifically, they draw constructs from the "family strengths" literature to examine the development of adolescents from three contemporary U.S. samples. They also assess the implications of family processes for children's development prospectively, as two of the three databases available for analysis contain longitudinal data. In addition, sub-group differences are examined. Thus, we have gone beyond correlating race and family structure with child outcomes to examine within sub-groups the usefulness of family process measures in explaining children's development. In addition, these analyses employ relatively large, nationally representative samples, elevating our certainty that the results can be extrapolated to the larger society.

FAMILY STRENGTHS RESEARCH

Over the years, a number of researchers and writers have focussed on positive family processes and child outcomes. For example, Hill (1971) and Gary (1983) have described the strengths of black families. Moreover, a substantial literature is developing that examines the factors that underlie successful development among *vulnerable* or *at risk* youth (Connell, Spencer, & Aber, 1993; Luther, 1991; Luther & Zigler, 1991; Dubow & Luster, 1990; Garmezy, 1985; Werner & Smith, 1982). Similarly, the *family strengths* literature has emphasized those positive processes that foster the well-being of children and adults as well.

A weakness of these literatures has been the lack of studies employing representative samples. Strong families have been identified, for example, by nominations from parish priests or local ministers and have tended to be white and middle class (Krysan, Moore & Zill, 1990). Nevertheless, a set of intuitively appealing constructs has been identified, some of which (e.g., communication) overlap with constructs identified from other perspectives. For example, the successful families described by the strong families literature shares many features with the authoritative families described by Baumrind (1971), as families in which parents are warm and caring and who discuss issues and reason with their children. The constructs employed in the family strengths literature to define a successful family include:

communication
encouragement of individuals
appreciation
religiosity or spirituality
time together
adaptability
clear roles
commitment to family
social connectedness

The purpose of the present project is to examine the utility of these *family strength* constructs as predictors of adolescent behavior problems. We approach this task cautiously, because even our initial perusal of the data indicated that the family process measures available in these national databases are somewhat limited. Moreover, none of the databases were designed to specifically measure family strengths. Consequently, our capacity to truly test the utility of this paradigm is inherently limited. Nevertheless, testing the constructs, insofar as is possible, is an important task because complete explanatory models of child development must include measures of family process as well as measures of socioeconomic status and social context. In fact, understanding the factors that foster development in all types of families can provide insights into actions and interaction patterns that families can use to strengthen their socialization practices despite inadequate economic resources. Thus, the aim of these analyses is to assess both the utility of these constructs and also the utility of the available data, and to suggest ways that future data collection efforts might improve upon previous efforts.

Three databases were analyzed for this project. Each database contained somewhat different measures of family strengths and youth outcomes. A summary of the family process constructs assessed by each database is provided in Table 1.

While the specific measures varied from one database to another, Table 1 shows that it was possible to operationalize most of the family strengths constructs in each of the databases.

Results from each of these analyses are presented in separate papers. The purpose of this document is to summarize and synthesize the results of these analyses and provide direction for future research and data development. The three papers are:

Family Functioning and Adolescent Behavior Problems: An Analysis of the National Survey of Families and Households by Brett Brown, Ph.D.

Assessing Family Strengths in the National Longitudinal Survey of Youth - Child Supplement by Donna Ruane Morrison, Ph.D. and Dana Glei, M.A.

The Effect of Family Strengths on Youth Behavior: An Analysis of the National Survey of Children by Barbara Sugland, Sc.D.

TABLE 1. AVAILABILITY OF FAMILY STRENGTHS AND FAMILY PROCESS MEASURES ACROSS DATA SETS

Family Strengths Constructs	NSC	NSFH	NLSY-CS
Communication	√	—	√
Encouragement of individuals	—	—	—
Commitment to family	√	√	—
Religious orientation/training/attendance	√	√	√
Social connectedness	√	√	√
Ability to adapt	√	—	—
Expressing appreciation	√	—	√
Clear roles	√	√	√
Time together	√	√	√
Other Family Process Constructs	**NSC**	**NSFH**	**NLSY-CS**
Strong punishment/spanking	√	—	√
Mother-partner relationship satisfaction	—	—	√
Parental conflict	—	√	√
Parental agreement about child	—	—	√
Parental depression	—	√	—

The data sets used in these analyses are: The National Survey of Children (NSC); the National Survey of Families and Households (NSFH); and the National Longitudinal Survey of Youth - Child Supplement (NLSY-CS)

While each paper takes its own approach to the issue, several common questions are addressed.

Are the family strengths constructs appropriate for varied sub-groups of the U.S. population, including single and two-parent families, blacks and whites, and boys and girls? Are statistically robust measures of family strengths available for these varied groups? In particular, the validity, reliability and predictive utility of family strengths measures across varied family structures are assessed in all three databases.

Do the several measures of family strengths occur together? That is, does a single construct underlie the individual measures of family strengths, or are there clusters of constructs that characterize a strong family?

Are the measures of family strengths associated with positive outcomes for children? Which characteristics of strong families are more strongly correlated with problem behavior among children and adolescents?

Do measures of family strengths predict to child outcomes across varied population sub-groups? If there are statistically significant associations between family strengths indicators and children's behavior problems, are they attributable to sample sections? Do associations hold controlling for other social and economic characteristics of families?

What suggestions might be made for the better measurement of family strengths and family processes in future data collection efforts?

DATA

National Survey of Families and Households (NSFH). Data from the initial wave of the NSFH include 13,014 persons, among whom are over 2,300 households with adolescents between the ages of twelve and eighteen. In-person interviews were conducted with a randomly chosen adult; this person is the parent in the sub-sample examined here. Additional information was supplied by the spouse. A fairly rich array of family process data was obtained, along with measures of child outcomes. However, no data were obtained directly from the adolescent, so only the parent perspective is available. Only the 1987 data were available for these analyses; although data from the second wave completed in 1992-93 will be available early in 1994, the NSFH analyses presented here are cross-sectional.

Three outcome measures are examined in the NSFH: a measure of behavior problems comprised of difficult behavior and personality characteristics, such as being irritable or sad, fearful, and bullying; a measure of more serious behavior problems, such as being suspended/expelled, running away, in trouble with the police; and a scale measuring conflict between parent and child over the youth's dress, friends, money, school, et cetera.

Results obtained using this data base are reported in Table 2.

National Longitudinal Survey of Youth - Child Supplement (NLSY-CS). In this database, a large, nationally representative sample of youth who were aged 14-21 in 1979 has been augmented with child development data. The youth respondents have been surveyed since 1979, to obtain information about their education and labor market experiences. Beginning in 1986, surveys and assessments of children born to the female respondents have been conducted every other year. Data for the 1986, 1988, 1990 panels are used for children ages 6 to 14 in 1988.

Because this is a sample of children born to a cohort of females aged 21-28 in 1986, the children in the sample all were born to relatively young mothers. Hence, this is a rather disadvantaged sample, particularly the adolescents, whose mothers were quite young when the children were born.

A number of measures of family processes have been added to the NLSY as a part of the child supplement; however, these measures are less rich than those available in the NSFH or the National Survey of Children. The particular strength of this database for the current analyses is the fact that the surveys are obtained every other year, permitting a prospective analysis of prior family characteristics on later child outcomes. In addition, indicators of behavior problems were obtained from both the mother and from the child; since mothers may not be aware of all the activities of their adolescents, the availability of child reports represents a substantial asset for this database as well.

Three outcomes are also assessed on the NLSY-CS, one reported by the mother and two based on child reports. The parent-report measure is a 32-item scale developed by Zill and Peterson (Zill, 1990) based on earlier work by Achenbach,

TABLE 2. SUMMARY OF RESULTS OF MULTIPLE REGRESSION ANALYSES: FAMILY STRENGTHS, BACKGROUND CHARACTERISTICS AND YOUTH BEHAVIOR. NATIONAL SURVEY OF FAMILIES AND HOUSEHOLDS

	Direction of Association		
Independent Variable	Behavior Problems I	Behavior Problems II	Parent/Child Conflict
Family Friendship	0	0	0
Family Within 25 Miles	0	0	0
Church Involvement	0	+	0
Parental Involvement in Youth Organizations	+	0	0
Socialize Outside of Family	0	0	0
Parent-Child Time Together	+	+	0
Commitment to Family	0	+	0
Encourage Independence Among Children	+	0	+
Parental Depression	–	0	–
Two-biological Parent, High Conflict Family*	–	0	–
Step, High Conflict Family	–	–	–
Step, Low Conflict Family	–	–	0
Divorced/Separated Female Headed Family	–	–	–
Never Married Female Headed Family	0	–	0
Single Male Headed Family	0	–	–
Gender of Adolescent: Male	0	–	–
Age of Adolescent	0	–	+
Gender of Parent: Male	0	0	+
Age of Parent	+	0	+
Race/Ethnicity of Respondent:			
Black	+	+	0
Hispanic	0	0	0
Other	0	0	0
Total Family Income	+	0	0
Parental Education: High School +	0	0	–
Family Received Public Assistance	–	0	0
Number of Persons in Household	–	+	0

Key: "0" = no significant association. "+" = associated with fewer behavior problems; "–" = associated with more behavior problems (p <= .05).
*For family structure variables, the omitted comparison group is the two-biological parent, low conflict family.

Rutter, Kellam, Langner, and other researchers, that measures acting out behaviors, depressed/withdrawn behaviors, and distractable/hyperactive behavior. The second measure is a child-reported scale that includes behaviors such as lying, damaging property, skipping school, et cetera. The third measure is a self perception profile for children which summarizes the child's assessment of their own general self-worth and academic competence.

Results obtained using the National Longitudinal Survey of Youth - Child Supplement are reported in Table 3.

The National Survey of Children (NSC). Three waves of the NSC have been conducted, in 1976 when the children were 7-11, in 1981 when they were 11-16, and in 1987 when they were 18-22.

In each wave, both the parent and the child were interviewed, and in the first two waves a teacher was also interviewed. For the analyses reported here, baseline demographic and family strengths measures were taken from the second wave of data collection, and except for a wave 2 teacher report, youth outcome measures were taken from the third interview. Five child/youth outcomes are examined: a 32-item Behavior Problem Index (very similar to the version in the NLSY-CS), the CES-D depression scale, youth-reported scale measuring delinquent behaviors in the previous 12 months, youth-reported drug/alcohol/tobacco use in the past 12 months, and a teacher rating of the child's school behavior.

Results obtained with the National Survey of Children are reported in Table 4.

TABLE 3. SUMMARY OF RESULTS OF MULTIPLE REGRESSION ANALYSES: FAMILY STRENGTHS, BACKGROUND CHARACTERISTICS AND YOUTH BEHAVIOR. NATIONAL LONGITUDINAL SURVEY OF YOUTH AND CHILD SUPPLEMENT

	Ages 6 to 9	Ages 10 to 14	
	Mother-reported BPI (Table 19, Col. 4)	Mother-reported BPI (Table 20, Col. 4)	Child-reported Behavior Problems (Table 21, Col. 4)
Family Strengths			
Appreciation	–	0	–
Interviewer-evaluated communication	–	0	0
Family discussion of TV	0	–	–
Family outings	0	na	na
Social connectedness	0	0	0
Discussion of sex with parent(s)	na	0	0
Child's religious attendance	na	0	0
Discipline Measures			
Mother-reported rules and chores	0	0	0
Child spanked at least once in prior week	+	+	+
Mother-Partner Measures			
Relationship satisfaction	0	–	0
Conflict	0	+	0
Agreement about child	na	+	0
Communication	–	0	0

Note: Results are from OLS regression models, including all family strength measures available for each age group as well as the following controls: Child's sex, age and race ethnicity; birthweight in ounces; number of years spent in child care in the first three years of life; indicator of whether child has handicapping condition; child's BPI score in 1988; mother's educational attainment, age at interview and number of children; family income in 1988; percent of previous five years spent in poverty; indicators for whether parents are divorced/separated, deceased, and never married.

TABLE 4. SUMMARY OF RESULTS OF MULTIPLE REGRESSION ANALYSES: FAMILY STRENGTHS, BACKGROUND CHARACTERISTICS AND YOUTH BEHAVIOR. NATIONAL SURVEY OF CHILDREN WAVE III, (1987)

Independent Variable	Direction of Association				
	Behavior Problems	Depression	Teacher Rating of Behavior	Delinquency	Drug Use
Parent-Child Communication	+	+	+	+	+
Appreciation	0	0	0	0	0
Family Activities	0	0	0	0	0
Clear Roles	+	+	+	0	0
Parent-Parent Communication	–	–	0	–	0
Commitment to Marriage & Family	0	0	0	+	+
Social Connectedness	0	0	0	0	0
Religious Training	0	0	+	0	+
Family Adaptability	+	0	0	0	0
Rules & Chores	0	0	0	0	0
Strong Punishment	–	–	0	–	0
Single Parent Family	–	+	0	0	0
Race–Black	0	0	–	0	+
Gender–Male	0	0	–	–	0
Fam Income <=$15k	0	0	0	0	0
AFDC	–	0	0	0	0
Family Size 4+	+	–	0	0	0
Parent's Education <12 yrs	–	0	0	0	0
Fair/Poor Neighborhood	–	0	0	0	0
Marital Disruption	0	0	0	0	0
Mothers AFB <=19	0	0	–	0	0
Age 14+	–	–	0	0	–

Key: "0" = no statistically significant association; "+" = positive influence (i.e., an increase in family strengths is associated with less negative outcomes); "–" = negative influence (i.e., an increase in family strengths is associated with more negative child outcomes); significance is at the $p \leq 0.05$ level.

AFB = Age at first birth.

ASSESSMENT OF THE RELIABILITY OF THE FAMILY STRENGTHS MEASURES

Overall and Within Population Sub-Groups. Although none of these databases explicitly includes measures intended to tap "family strengths" constructs, it was generally possible to develop measures that assess many of these constructs with reasonable reliability. In most cases, only a few items were available to construct scales, reducing scale reliability; nevertheless, each database yielded a number of scales with adequate reliabilities. Other constructs had to be examined with single-term indicators, however; and some constructs could not be assessed at all, particularly with the NLSY-CS. These analyses clearly indicate that, if a particular family process is considered important to assess, multiple item scales need to be developed.

Moreover, before new scales are included in national surveys, the utility of the scale items should be assessed among varied socioeconomic and race/ethnic groups because the nature and importance of various constructs may differ for different types of families. For example, in our analysis of the NSFH, only among step-families and female headed families was the measure "encourages independence" associated with significantly fewer behavior problems; this may suggest either that encouraging independence has a different meaning in other family types or has different effects in other family types. Similarly, communication within the family requires different measures when there is one parent than when there are two, and the significance of social connectedness seems to differ across family types. However, the number of such instances is fairly modest: in general, the various family strengths do seem to be relevant to most family types.

In general, the distributions of mean scores on indicators of family strength suggest that such strengths are common among all families, regardless of family structure or race. When differences were noted, families containing both biological parents tend to have the more positive ranking, particularly on parent-report items; however, given substantial differences in socioeconomic status across the family sub-groups, the relatively minimal differences found in measures of family process could suggest common processes unrelated to income, race, and family structure. However, reliance on overly global measures that may miss differences that do exist could account for the lack of group differences.

Analyses generally indicate that measures of different family strength constructs are significantly and positively correlated with one another; however, the magnitudes of the correlations are generally quite modes. Furthermore, none of the factor analyses conducted on any of the databases indicated the presence of a single underlying construct that could be labelled a "family strength" scale. In fact, factor analyses, within the NSC, suggested several underlying family strengths domains, especially for single parent and minority females. Also, when data from multiple respondents was available, items provided by a given respondent were found to cluster together, suggesting that any given respondent has a unique perspective. This underscores the value of multiple respondents.

THE ASSOCIATION BETWEEN FAMILY STRENGTHS AND BEHAVIOR PROBLEMS

The most central question for these analyses is whether family strengths affect the incidence of problem behaviors in children and youth across all three data sets. Comparable outcome variables were defined across the several databases so that, insofar as is possible, the predictive utility of the family strength measures could be assessed.

Correlational analyses do indeed indicate that the presence of varied family strengths is associated with fewer behavior problems among children and youth almost without exception. For example, strong parent-child communication, joint activities, and clear and consistent expectations were all associated with fewer subsequent behavior problems among young adults in the NSC. Similarly, in the NLSY-CS, measures of appreciation, communication, family outings, and social connectedness all predict to fewer subsequent behavior problems among school-aged children. The magnitude and level of significance of the associations varies, and sometimes associations are not statistically significant; but the direction of the effect rarely goes opposite to prediction. That is, the data virtually never suggest that the presence of family strengths is correlated with the more frequent occurrence of behavior problems. (One example of an exception is several correlations in the NSFH analyses, where socializing with neighbors and friends has a small, but positive, association with the frequency of adolescent behavior problems.) Measures of harsh or strong punishment, marital conflict, and parent-child conflict, on the other hand, do predict later problems.

These correlations provide clear evidence that family strengths are associated with child outcomes; specifically, with fewer child behavior problems. However, they do not address the very important question of whether these correlations remain when family background differences are taken into account. Multivariate analyses were therefore conducted on each of the databases to address this question.

MULTIVARIATE MODELS OF FAMILY STRENGTHS AND BEHAVIOR PROBLEMS

Controlling for socioeconomic variables, such as parental education, income, race, and family structure, tends to diminish but not erase the effects of family process variables. In general, the family functioning measures continue to have small but significant effects on child and adolescent behavior problems, even after controls for social and demographic variables were included in multivariate models.

In the NSC, parent-child communication is the one family strength that demonstrates a significant influence on all five of the youth outcomes examined, net of background factors. Clear roles also predict to more positive youth outcomes on three of the five measures of behavior problems, while commitment to family and religious training have positive effects on two outcomes, net of control variables in this database. Parent-parent communication, interestingly, predicts to more problems on three of the five child outcomes. Whether this reflects parents who are preoccupied with each other rather than the child, or reflects instead intense parental communication in response to child behavior problems that are already developing at the time of the 1981 interview, is not clear. This ambiguity does suggest, however, the importance of knowing not just that communication has occurred but something about the content of that communication. On the other hand, a number of the family strength measures do not predict to any of the behavior problem measures in multivariate models, including appreciation, social connectedness, and family activities.

In the NLSY-CS, the family strength measures have little effect on child outcomes once socioeconomic variables are controlled. In fact, none of the family strength measures consistently affect children's behavior and self-perceptions, though appreciation is important in a number of models. Affection and communication also appear to be promising constructs; but the measures of family

processes in the NLSY-CS are quite weak. The lack of effects may reflect the paucity of strong measures of family processes or the limited variability found in the disadvantaged sample of NLSY-CS mothers with school-aged children. Since a goal of examining family strengths, however, is to identify family processes that represent a positive resource for families regardless of their socioeconomic assets, the minimal effects in this sample are important to recognize.

In the NSFH, the family strength variables found to be the most important are those which tap the internal family processes, including parent-child time together, parental commitment to the family, and parental encouragement of independence in the child. The availability of extended family members and family involvement in the community are not found to predict directly to child outcomes in the multivariate models. The effects of involvement in church and family involvement in the community organizations are minimal once other variables are controlled. This pattern suggests, at most, an indirect effect of such variables. Perhaps, for example, external factors such as extended family involvement may affect internal factors such as parent-child time together, and thus, affect the child. Hence, external factors that influence more proximal influences could indirectly affect the child outcomes assessed here.

Some of the variables available in the three databases analyzed are not technically a part of the family strengths tradition but represent constructs that have nevertheless been found in other studies to affect children's development. In order to explore the expectation that the family strengths measures did not fully tap all dimensions of family functioning, several of these measures are included in the multivariate models not only as control variables, but also as substantive variables. These variables include measures of harsh punishment and family and marital conflict. These measures are included along with socioeconomic controls and are found to have strong negative effects on children's development, net of background factors and measures of family strengths. For example, in the NLSY-CS, though family strength variables are not significant in multivariate analyses, the use of spanking by the parent to discipline their school-aged child predicts to subsequent behavior problems. Another negative indicator is that of parental depression. The NSFH contains a revised version of the CES-D depression scale. Higher parental depression is found strongly associated with poorer child outcomes among two biological parent families. Analyses of the NSFH indicate that family functioning measures may be as important as socio-demographic variables in explaining behavior problems. For two of the three NSFH outcomes, adding the full set of family process variables is associated with a near doubling of the variance explained.

A potential problem even with the multivariate models is that many of the family strengths measures, as operationalized in these databases, may be confounded with family structure. For example, child-related activities and communication may be affected by the number of adults present in the family and their relationship to the child. Moreover, membership in particular family structure categories, such as single parent families, is correlated with attributes such as low parental education and low incomes. To examine the possibility that such selectivity factors are distorting the multivariate results, models are estimated on NLSY-CS data employing selection models (Maddala, 1983) that take both observable and unobservable in differences between the groups into account. First, a probit model is estimated predicting membership in a continuously married family compared to membership in any other family type. The Inverse Mills Ratio derived from this estimation, the hazard instrument, is then included in the multivariate equation predicting child behavior problems. Results from this equation are found to be about the same as the estimates without controlling for selectivity, both in terms of magnitude and statistical significance. Hence, sample selectivity is not found to be a significant problem for these analyses.

DISCUSSION AND CONCLUSIONS

Overall, the results from these analyses suggest that including measures of family processes, such as family strengths constructs, in large-scale national surveys is promising. Measures of family processes predict to later behavior problems even when social and economic variables are controlled. Results suggest that parent-child interaction in particular (such as parent-child communication) can affect children's behavior over and above the influence of income, family structure, race, and parent education. Moreover, family process measures seem to be important within subgroups defined by family structure and race, as well as in the total sample.

However, the variance explained by family strength variables is quite modest. Several factors may explain the minimal associations found here. The primary reason probably reflects the lack of theoretical or conceptual framework for the family strengths measures. The constructs were developed and refined by researchers and practitioners who tended to first identify successful families and then to identify the characteristics of those families. This process yielded an intuitively meaningful set of family strengths in need of theoretical linkage with the child development and family sociology literatures. Overlaps exist with Coleman's theory of social capital (Coleman, 1988), research on resilient or invulnerable children (Luther, 1991; Dubow & Luster, 1990; Garmezy, 1985), studies of successful development among at-risk children (Sugland & Hyatt, 1993; Sugland, Blumenthal, & Hyatt, 1993), studies of strong black families (Hill, 1971; Gary et. al., 1983), and child development theories such as the parenting paradigm proposal by Baumrind (1971).

A strong linkage between the insights afforded by the successful families literature and the theoretical perspectives of these other traditions would help identify the gaps on the list of family processes identified in the family strengths literature. For example, one critical role that families may play that is not considered in the family strengths constructs is how parents direct their children into peer activities and friendships. We know that peers play an increasingly important role in children's behavior as they move into the teen years, yet the role of parents in the unfolding of that process has not been the focus of much research.

A stronger theoretical approach to the development of family strengths constructs would also inform hypotheses regarding which family strengths are important as direct effects and which function indirectly. For example, the effect of religion on children may be transmitted indirectly through family structure or commitment to marriage, or it may function as a direct effect on the child's own standards and values. In addition, theory would inform hypotheses about which family strength constructs, if any, are redundant. For example, are parent-child activities, family religious activities, and religiosity discrete constructs, or do they overlap in part? Similarly, some variables may be important primarily in interaction with other variables. For example, the importance of extended kin may be manifest primarily among single parent families, where they play an essential role supporting the childbearing efforts of a solo parent.

Clear theoretical arguments indicating the mediating mechanisms between constructs and child outcomes are needed more generally. For example, what is it about parent-child communication, family religiosity, and interaction with extended family members and friends that is hypothesized to foster positive child development? Specification of these mediating hypotheses would enable the construction of survey items more likely to assess the intended concept. Thus, to assess the role of parent-child communication, for example, it is necessary to specify whether the construct should be the quantity of communication per se, the occurrence or communication on particular topics such as drugs or behavior, the style of communication, or simply whether the child feels he or she could communicate with his or her parents if a need arose.

Apart from insufficient theoretical development, the family strengths constructs lack adequate measurement in existing national surveys. Indeed, this critique would have to be extended more generally to most measures of family processes in current national surveys. Minimal resources have been devoted to developing scales appropriate for survey administration. Complex, multi-faceted constructs such as communication and spirituality are often measured with a single item. Moreover, the validity of items and scales and their underlying constructs in different sub-populations has not been assessed. The role of the extended family and religious institutions, for example, may be quite different in black and single parent families than in white or two biological parent families. Similarly, communication within the family requires different measures when there is one parent than when there are two, and the significance of social connectedness seems to differ across family types. However, the number of such instances where a construct is relevant for *only* one family type is fairly modest: in general, the various family strengths constructs do seem to be relevant to most family types. The need is for development of scale items appropriate in varied types of families which will create more valid and reliable scales. To fully understand the role of family processes apart from family socioeconomic resources in shaping the development of children will require an investment in measure development.

These analyses have also underscored the importance of multiple respondents. In particular, obtaining the perspective of the child or youth on family processes and on their own behavior seems to be essential. In addition, the importance of nationally representative longitudinal data has been highlighted in these analyses. To be able to extrapolate findings, representative samples are necessary. To begin to understand causality, longitudinal data are essential. Narrow studies of delimited populations are very helpful for developing constructs and measures. Eventually, however, it is necessary to assess promising constructs with representative data and to test the predictive power of the constructs with longitudinal data.

Ultimately, the value of the present analyses is their systematic examination of promising constructs developed in a particular literature—(family strengths)—using stringent multivariate methods. This interplay across disciplines and methods can enhance our understanding of the processes that underlie child and adolescent development much more rapidly than if narrow specialties work in isolation. These analyses indicate that most of the family strength constructs do affect the development of children and adolescents, net of socioeconomic variables and across varied social groups. At the same time, they indicate a need for theory-driven reliable measures, scale items that are appropriate within varied cultural groups and within different family structures, and variables that assess the critical mediating processes that connect parental inputs with child outcomes.

REFERENCES

Administration for Children and Families. (1993). *Characteristics and financial circumstances of AFDC recipients.* Washington, DC: U.S. Department of Health and Human Services.

Baumrind, D. (1971). Current patterns of parental authority. *Developmental Psychology Monographs, 4*(1, Part 2).

Bumpass, L., & Rindfuss, R. R. (1979). Children's experience of marital disruption. *American Journal of Sociology, 85*(1):49-65.

Coleman, J. (1988). Social capital in the creation of human capital. *American Journal of Sociology. (94)*:595-5120.

Connell, J. P., Spencer, M. B., & Aber, J. (1993). *Risk and resilience in African-American youth: Context, self action and outcomes in school.* Philadelphia: Public/Private Ventures.

Dubow, E. F., & Luster, T. (1990). Adjustment of children born to teenage mothers: The contribution of risk and protective factors. *Journal of Marriage and the Family, 52*, 393-404.

Garmezy, N. (1985). Stress-resistant children: The search for protective factors. In J. E. Stevenson, (Ed.), *Recent research in development psychopathology,* Chapter 19, pp. 213-233. Oxford: Pergamon Press.

Gary, L. E., Beatty, L. A., Berry, G. L. et. al. (1983). *Stable black families: Final report*. Washington, DC: Mental Health Research and Development Center, Institute for Urban Affairs and Research, Howard University.

Hill, R. B. (1971). *The strength of black families*. New York: Independence Publishers Group.

Luther, S. S. (1991). Vulnerability and resilience: A study of high risk adolescents. *Child Development, 62,* 600-616.

Luther, S. S., & Zigler, E. (1991). Vulnerability and competence: A review of research on resilience in childhood. *American Journal of Orthopsychology, 61*(1):6-22.

National Center for Health Statistics. (1993). Advance report of final natality statistics, 1990. *Monthly Vital Statistics Report,* 41(9):suppl. Hyattsville, MD: Public Health Service.

Sugland, B., & Hyatt, B. (forthcoming). *Social capital and the ordering of life events among "at-risk" young women.* Washington, DC: Child Trends, Inc.

Sugland, B., Blumenthal, C., & Hyatt, B. (forthcoming). *Successful life events among "at-risk" young women: The mediating effect of social capital.* Washington, DC: Child Trends, Inc.

Werner, E. E., Bierman, J. M., & French, F. E. (1971). *The children of Kauai: A longitudinal study from the prenatal period to age ten.* Honolulu: University of Hawaii Press.

EDWARD ANTHONY, PH.D.,
Director
Policy and Planning Offices of Special Education
and Rehabilitation Services
U.S. Department of Education

Summary

Dr. Nick Zill's paper gave an overview of the current state of family data and databases. Systematic review methodology and describing mechanisms for synthesizing family research was discussed by Dr. John Lyons. Responses were made by Drs. Ron Haskins and Kristin Moore. Dr. Moore's paper dealt with the strengths in families and Dr. Haskin discussed health data and its role in research and policy.

Participants emphasized the need for compact sets of questions to measure and describe family processes. These questions need to be consistent across surveys to insure consistent measurements and analysis. This requires good survey design, which is itself a complicated process.

Dr. Zill believes we need to develop better measurement instruments within federal statistical agencies to insure better test validity. Although there have been many measurement scales designed, more research is needed to further refine the art of collecting the maximum amount of data with the fewest questions. Dr. Haskins emphasized the need to simplify the complex issues so that congressional staffers can understand them and, hopefully, influence the decisions of congress members.

Some participants stressed the need to find out more about labor force participation. This is an important element in measuring family health, yet data gathering techniques in this area are crude.

Panelists also voiced concern about accurate collection of participation data, especially for program evaluation purposes.

The timeliness of data was discussed. Dr. Haskins felt good data that can be replicated and is agreed upon by experts in the field is the most important issue. Dr. Zill argued that timeliness is important and technology has made that possible, but it requires huge financial resources.

Two methodological problems with regard to family research were raised: 1) the problem with the single respondent method of surveying and 2) linear models are not sophisticated enough to illustrate the complexity of family research.

DAVID H. OLSON, PH.D.
Professor, Family Social Science
University of Minnesota

JUDY WATSON TIESEL
University of Minnesota

Assessment of Family Functioning

This is a chapter in the book by Bruce Rounsav-ille (Ed.). (In press). Diagnostic Sourcebook. *Washington, DC: National Institute on Drug Abuse (NIDA).*

Effective assessment of family functioning has improved dramatically in the last decade in terms of reliability, validity, and clinical utility (Grotevant & Carlson, 1989; Touliatos et al., 1990). Family inventories provide a critical bridge between research, theory and practice (Olson, 1976). Also, the effective interplay of research, theory and practice facilitates the advancement of each domain.

Theoretical advancements in the family field have been retarded by a lack of effective family assessment instruments. However, in the last few years considerable work has been done and a variety of self-report inventories has been developed (Fredman & Sherman, 1987; Grotevant & Carlson, 1989; Jacob & Tennenbaum, 1988). Concern about the reliability, validity and clinical utility of these instruments has also been growing. The traditional psychometric procedures are increasingly being used to improve these inventories.

An important assessment issue in the family field is whether the data are collected from the "insider's perspective" or from the "outsider's perspective" (Olson, 1977). While self-reports can provide information on how family members perceive their family functioning (insider's perspective), behavioral and observational assessments are required to provide the outsider's perspective.

Research and clinical work have demonstrated consistently that these two perspectives provide different and often conflicting sources of information (Olson, 1985). This could be because families are unable to accurately report what they either do not want to see or have not been trained to see, such as systemic interaction. On the other hand, it could be because outside observers are unable to understand the shared meanings that a family has developed (Grotevant & Carlson, 1989). While it was assumed initially that one approach is more valid than the other, it is more appropriate to consider *both* perspectives as relevant and necessary for a comprehensive assessment of marital and family functioning (Olson, 1985).

This review will focus exclusively on self-report family assessment and will build on the earlier reviews of these inventories by both the authors and other scholars in the field (Fredman & Sherman, 1987; Grotevant & Carlson, 1989; Jacob & Tennenbaum, 1988; Touliatos, Perlmutter & Straus, 1990). Four of the five self-report instruments selected also have a behavioral rating scale which can be used for assessment. Even though the dimensions of each self-report scale match those of the rating scales, attempts have not been consistent to assess the level of agreement across these two methodological approaches. Often the behavioral rating scales have not undergone the same rigorous development used for the self-report measures. For a more comprehensive review of a range of observational measures, see Markman and Notarius (1987) and Grotevant and Carlson (1989).

The five family self-report inventories selected for this more in-depth review represent those that met the following two criteria. First, they each tapped relevant theoretical dimensions that are generally agreed to be important theoretically and clinically. Second, these five inventories are the most highly developed psychometrically; investigators have attempted to continually improve the reliability, validity and clinical utility of the scales.

Specifically, the five inventories selected for this review are, in *alphabetical* order: (1) *Family Adaptability and Cohesion Evaluation Scales: FACES II*, developed by Olson, Portner, and Bell (1982), and *FACES III*, developed by Olson, Portner, and Lavee (1985), (2) *Family Assessment Device (FAD)* constructed by Epstein, Baldwin, and Bishop (1983), (3) *Family Assessment Measure (FAM III)* developed by Skinner, Steinhauer, and Santa-Barbara (1984), (4) *Family Environment Scale (FES)* developed by Moos and Moos (1981), and (5) *Self-Report Family Inventory (SRI)* developed by Hulgus, Hampson, and Beavers (1985). The publisher or source for purchasing these inventories is indicated in Appendix A.

THEORETICAL DIMENSIONS UTILIZED BY THESE
FIVE FAMILY INVENTORIES

Review of both the family therapy literature and theoretical frameworks in the family and other social science fields has revealed the salience of at least *three dimensions* for understanding family functioning and dynamics. These are: *cohesion* (togetherness), *adaptability* (change), and *communication* (Olson et al., 1979; Olson et al., 1980; Olson et al., 1989).

Table 1 indicates the theoretical dimensions of cohesion, adaptability, and communication, and how the specific scales in each of these five instruments relate to these three dimensions.

Since Family Adaptability and Cohesion Evaluation Scales (FACES) was built on a theoretical review of the literature, the primary dimensions assessed in FACES are cohesion and adaptability. Separate scales have been developed to assess marital communication (Olson et al., 1982) and

parent-adolescent communication (Barnes & Olson, 1982, 1985). In the Family Assessment Device (FAD), affective involvement taps the cohesion dimension; behavior control, problem-solving, and roles tap the adaptability dimension; and communication and affective responsiveness relate to the communication dimension. For the Family Assessment Measure (FAM III), the concepts and scales are very similar to the FAD scales. More specifically, affective involvement taps the cohesion dimension, while task performance, role performance, and control tap the adaptability dimension. Communication and affective expression relate to the communication dimension. Values and norms are the only subscales that do not seem to fit into the three dimensions.

In the Family Environment Scale (FES), the cohesion and independence scales relate to the cohesion dimension; the control and organizational scales relate to adaptability; and the expressiveness and conflict scales relate to the communication dimension. In the FES, there are four additional scales that do not fit into these categories; they are achievement orientation, active-recreational orientation, intellectual-cultural orientation, and moral-religious emphasis.

In the Self-report Family Inventory (SFI), cohesion is tapped by the subscales of positive emotional expression and cohesion. Leadership relates to the adaptability dimension, and the communication and conflict resolution subscales relate to the communication dimension. The family health scale is an overall measure consisting of items both unique and borrowed from the other subscales.

CRITERIA FOR EVALUATING FAMILY
ASSESSMENT INVENTORIES

In order to provide a systematic framework for evaluating these five family assessment scales, a set of criteria was developed and used (Table 2). The theoretical domain and model which provide the foundation for the scale were considered very important. Next, the assessment level dealt with whether the family as a whole was evaluated or whether the instrument also considered the component parts (i.e., dyadic and individual level functioning). The number of scales and items were considered along with the normative sample and whether clinical samples had been collected. Finally, because of the increasing awareness in the family field of the importance of ethnic diversity

Table 1

Five Family Inventories Related to Three Theoretical Dimensions

Inventory	Cohesion	Adaptability	Communication	Other
Family Adaptability & Cohesion Evaluation Scales (FACES III)	• Cohesion	• Adaptability	*Marital Communication *Parent-Adolescent Communication	
Family Assessment Device (FAD)	• Affective Involvement	• Problem Solving • Behavior Control • Roles	• Communication • Affective Responsiveness	
Family Assessment Measure (FAM III)	• Affective Involvement	• Task Accomplish-ment • Control • Role Performance	• Communication • Affective Expression	• Values and Norms
Family Environment Scale (FES)	• Cohesion • Independence	• Organization • Control	• Expressiveness • Conflict	• Achievement • Active-Recreational • Moral Religious • Intellectual-Cultural
Self-report Family Inventory (SFI)	• Positive Emotional Expression • Cohesion	• Leadership	• Communication • Conflict Resolution	• Family Health

These inventories are available from David Olson and are printed in the Family Inventories Manual Olson et al., 1985)

TABLE 2: CRITERIA FOR EVALUATING FAMILY
ASSESSMENT SCALES

Theoretical Domain and Model
Assessment Level (Individual, Couple or Family)
Number of Scales, Number of Items
Availability of Norms

Reliability:
Internal Consistency Reliability
Test-Retest Reliability

Validity:
Face and Content Validity
Correlation Between Scales in Instrument
Correlation with Social Desirability
Concurrent Validity
Correlation Between Family Members
Discrimination Validity

Clinical Utility:
Usefulness of Self-report Scale
Ease of Administration and Scoring
Clinical Rating Scale
Applicability to Ethnic Diversity Issues

issues, each scale was evaluated to see how such issues were addressed (Table 2).

Reliability focused on the internal consistency of the scale. This assessed the degree of relationship between the items in the scale. Scales with high levels of homogeneity, as measured by Cronbach's alpha, indicated good *internal consistency reliability*. If the reliability is too high, it could indicate that the items are too similar, and this could reduce the content validity because the items only tap a limited range of issues. *Test-retest reliability* assessed the stability of the scores over a period of time. Short-term reliability was often over two to six weeks, with the long-term reliability extending from six to twelve months.

The validity of these scales was assessed in various ways. Basically, validity assesses whether the scale measures what it proports to measure. *Face validity* assesses whether the final instrument "looks like" it measures what it is intended to measure. Judgments about the adequacy of the items are often made by "experts" in a content area.

Content validity assesses whether there is a good representative sample of the range of content issues related to that domain. Empirically, it can be assessed by determining whether the items seem to fit together conceptually. Factor analysis can be used to demonstrate this by determining whether the items load on a particular factor.

Another approach for assessing the content validity of an instrument is to determine the correlation between the various scales or subscales within the same instrument. The correlation of the scales with social desirability is particularly problematic with self-report scales. Therefore, it is useful in developing scales to assess this correlation and attempt to minimize a scale's correlation with social desirability.

Concurrent validity is the extent to which the scale correlates with other scales that measure the same construct (Campbell & Fiske, 1959). This is assessed by comparing a scale with others intended to measure the same construct.

The correlation between responses of family members is one area that should be considered. Currently, considerable evidence points to a lack of agreement between family members and self-report scales that measure family dynamics. Lastly, discriminating between normal and problem families is one important criterion for assessing the discriminant validity of the scales.

In considering the clinical utility of these scales, it is important to consider how useful the scale is clinically and how difficult it is to administer and score. Those investigators who developed the self-report scales also developed a *clinical rating scale* which can be used by therapists or raters to evaluate the behavior of family members, either in therapy or in some observational situation. This type of clinical rating scale provides an outsider perspective which can be compared with the self-report descriptions (insider's perspective) provided by family members. Currently, most existing research indicates a lack of congruence between these insider and outsider perspectives, even within the same theoretical model (Olson, 1985).

The following five self-report scales are presented in *alphabetical* order.

1. FAMILY ADAPTABILITY AND COHESION EVALUATION SCALES (FACES)

Theoretical Domain

The Family Adaptability and Cohesion Evaluation Scales (FACES) has undergone three revisions in an effort to assess the two major dimensions of the Circumplex Model, i.e., cohesion and adaptability. Cohesion is defined as the emotional bonding that individuals in the family have toward each other. Adaptability relates to family power structures, role relationships and relationship rules (Table 3).

The Circumplex Model was developed by Olson, Russell, and Sprenkle (1980, 1983, 1989) in

Cohesion	Cohesion is the degree of emotional bonding between family members.
Adaptability	The ability of a marital and family system to change its power structure, role relationships, and relationship rules in response to situational and developmental stress.

an attempt to construct a model that would help bridge research, theory and practice. Communication, the third dimension of the Circumplex Model, facilitates movement on the other two dimensions. These three dimensions were derived from a conceptual clustering of numerous concepts in the marriage and family field (Olson et al., 1983).

An essential characteristic of the Circumplex Model is its curvilinear relationship with family functioning. Extreme levels of cohesion or adaptability represent Extreme family types and are more problematic than moderate levels which represent Balanced family types. The observational measure, the *Clinical Rating Scale (CRS)*, has continued to support the curvilinear hypothesis (Thomas & Olson, 1991).

A recent theoretical update (Olson, 1991) indicated that FACES II and III operate in a *linear manner*, a phenomenon due to the nature of the self-report scales, not the underlying theoretical model. Hence, a 3-D Circumplex Model was introduced in which high FACES scores represent Balanced types, and low scores represent Extreme types. A fourth version of FACES is currently in progress and is designed to measure the curvilinearity of the Circumplex Model.

Reliability and Validity

The normative sample for FACES II was 2,453 adults from across the life cycle and 412 adolescents. FACES III, the most recent version, has been used in over 500 research projects with good evidence of reliability and validity. Recently, however, some findings have suggested that FACES II has some advantages over FACES III. The alpha reliability is higher in the 30-item FACES II than in the 20-item FACES III. The test-retest reliability for FACES II was relatively high, .83 for cohesion and .80 for adaptability over a four to five week period.

The face and content validity of the scale are generally very good. In terms of validity, FACES III may have some advantages over FACES II. The correlation between adaptability and cohesion is considerably higher in FACES II (.65) compared to FACES III (.03). Social desirability responses remained approximately the same across FACES II and III when correlated with cohesion (.39 and .35, respectively). For adaptability, the correlation with social desirability was reduced from .38 in FACES II to virtually nothing in FACES III.

However, the concurrent validity for FACES II is higher than for FACES III, especially for family adaptability. That is, other instruments which measure constructs similar to cohesion and adaptability correlate higher with FACES II than FACES III (Green 1989; Hampson et al., 1991).

Considerable evidence indicates that FACES discriminates between clinical groups. Most past research has focused on distinguishing between Balanced versus Extreme types in the Circumplex Model. The FACES manual cites many studies which used either of the first two versions to successfully discriminate between clinical/high risk families and balanced/control groups. FACES as a linear measure can distinguish balanced, mid-range and extreme family types. Recent evidence also demonstrates the value of the Clinical Rating Scale (CRS) in discriminating problem from "non-problem" families (Thomas & Olson, 1991).

Clinical Utility

The clinical utility of FACES is very good. It takes approximately ten to fifteen minutes to complete the scale, and children from ages 10-12 can be administered FACES since it is written at a seventh grade reading level.

As mentioned, the observational measure, Clinical Rating Scale (CRS), has been designed to be used independently or in conjunction with FACES. In addition to adaptability and cohesion, it also assesses the communication dimension.

Many studies have tested the effectiveness of using FACES with ethnic populations. To date, research has been done with Mexican-American, Puerto Rican, African-American, Chinese-American, and multi-ethnic family samples with very good results. Currently, work is underway to establish norms for various ethnic groups (Table 4).

2. FAMILY ASSESSMENT DEVICE (FAD)

Theoretical Domain

The Family Assessment Device (FAD) is based on the McMaster Model of Family Functioning

Table 4

FACES Criteria

	Family Adaptability & Cohesion Evaluation Scales (FACES)	
<u>Theoretical Domain and Model</u>	Family System Circumplex Model	
<u>Assessment Level</u>	Family as Whole	
<u>Norms</u> Normative Sample Clinical	n = 2,453 Adults Across Life Cycle Problem Families Chemically Dependent	
	FACES II	FACES III
<u>Number of Scales and Items</u>	2 Scales; 30 Items total 16 Cohesion Items 14 Adaptability Items	2 Scales; 20 Items total 10 Cohesion Items 10 Adaptability Items
<u>Reliability</u> Internal Consistency	Very good evidence Cohesion (r = .87) Adaptability (r = .78)	Good evidence Cohesion (r = .77) Adaptability (r = −.62)
Test-Retest	FACES II (4–5 weeks) .83 for Cohesion .80 for Adaptability	
<u>Validity</u> Face Validity		Very good evidence
Content Validity		Very good evidence
Correlation Between Scales	Cohesion & Adaptibility (r = .65)	Cohesion & Adaptibility (r = .03)
Correlation with Social Desirability	Cohesion & SD (r = .39) Adaptability & SD (r = .38)	Cohesion & SD (r = .39) Adaptability & SD (r = .00)
Concurrent Validity	Good evidence (linear relationship)	Good evidence (linear relationship)
Correlation Between Family Members		X = H/W/A (n = 370) Cohesion (r = .42) Adaptability (r = .20)
Discrimination Between Groups		Very good evidence
<u>Clinical Utility</u> Usefulness of Self-report Scale Ease of Administering and Scoring Clinical Rating Scale Ethnic Diversity Utility	Very good evidence Very easy Yes Good evidence	

TABLE 5: FAMILY ASSESSMENT DEVICE (FAD)

Affective Involvement	The degree to which the family as a whole shows interest in the values and activities of individual family members.
Behavioral Control	The pattern the family adopts in handling physically dangerous situations, meeting and expressing psychobiological needs and dealing with interpersonal socializing behavior. Four styles of control are described: (1) rigid, (2) flexible, (3) laissez-faire, and (4) chaotic.
Roles	Roles of the recurrent patterns of behavior by which individuals fulfill family functions. The necessary family roles include provision of resources, nurturance and support, sexual gratification, life skills development, and maintenance and management of the family systems.
Problem Solving	The family's ability to resolve problems, both instrumental and affective types, in a way that maintains affective family functioning. The problem-solving process is broken down into seven stages.
Communication	Communication is defined as the exchange of information within a family. Communication is focused on the verbal level and is subdivided into instrumental and affective areas. Two independent dimensions of communication are emphasized: (1) clear vs. masked, (2) direct vs. indirect. Pairing these two styles identifies four patterns of communication.
Affective Responsiveness	This is the ability of family to respond to a range of issues with appropriate quality and quantity of feelings. Regarding quality, the concern is whether there is a full range of feelings expressed and whether the emotion is consonant with the situation.

developed by Epstein and colleagues (1983). The FAD assesses the family as a whole with emphasis on current family functioning. The McMaster Model of Family Functioning is based on the earlier conceptual framework of the Family Categories Schema (Epstein et al., 1968) which was originally developed and used in a study of 110 "nonclinical" families (Westley & Epstein, 1969). In addition to a general functioning scale, there are six theoretical dimensions which are built into the FAD instrument. The conceptual dimensions are affective involvement, behavioral control, roles, problem solving, communication, and affective responsiveness. Conceptual definitions of these scales are provided in Table 5.

Reliability and Validity

The norms for the FAD are based on 503 adults (Epstein & Bishop, 1981). The internal consistency reliability of the seven FAD scales generally is very good. The mean reliability is .78; the range for the seven scales is .72 to .92. The test-retest reliability over a one-week period also was relatively good with a mean of .70 and a range of .66 to .75 (n = 53).

A more recent study (Kabacoff et al., 1990) investigating reliability from data obtained from the FAD research files found the strongest internal reliability for the General Functioning subscale (.83 for the nonclinical group), while the Roles subscale had only marginal reliability of .57.

Both face validity and content validity of the scales appear very good.

One of the more problematic issues with the FAD is the high correlation between the seven scales (mean = .56, range = .37 to .76). This occurs primarily because of the high correlation with the global scale of General Functioning. When partial correlations were used to hold General Functioning constant, correlations between the scales dropped to an average of .11.

A series of studies examining the reliability and validity of the FAD (Miller et al., 1985) found that the correlations of the scales with social desirability ranged from −.06 to −.19 (n = 164). Concurrent validity was examined in this project by comparing with two other family scales, FACES II and Family Unit Inventory. The obtained correlations were generally quite good and congruent with theoretical expectations, and the relationship between FAD and FACES II was linear.

In terms of discriminative validity, two studies showed good evidence of the ability to distinguish between clinical and nonclinical samples. In the first study (Epstein & Bishop, 1981), a sample of 218 nonclinical individuals was compared with a sample of 98 clinical individuals. There were significant differences between groups on all of the scales. By using discriminant analysis, they were able to predict to some extent whether a family came from a clinical (64% accuracy) or nonclinical (76% accuracy) group.

In a second discriminative validity study (Miller et al., 1985), 42 clinical patients were assessed by family therapists and rated for healthy or unhealthy family functioning on each of the six dimensions. At the same time, all family members completed an FAD. Results indicated that the FAD scores corresponded to the clinicians' assessments on every dimension except Behavior Control. These results along with theoretical support were then used to establish cut-off scores to differentiate healthy from unhealthy families on each dimension, with a fairly good rate of success in the following: sensitivity (57-83%), specificity (64-79%), and diagnostic confidence (68-89%).

More recently, the General Functioning (GF) subscale was tested for reliability and validity in an Ontario child health study (Byles et al., 1988). This 12-item scale, when used in a sample of 1,869, resulted in very good alpha reliability (.86). Validity was assessed by hypothesizing relationships between criterion variables within the data set and the GF scale. All findings were in the predicted direction, except for socioeconomic status and family structure, which were weakly related.

Clinical Utility

The clinical utility of the FAD appears to be very good. A number of articles have been written on the McMaster Model in clinical treatment and training (e.g., Bishop & Epstein, 1985; Bishop & Epstein, 1987; Epstein, Keitner, Bishop, & Miller, 1988; Keitner, 1990). It appears to be a clinically useful scale that is easy to score and can be used with children down to the age of 12.

There is also a McMaster Clinical Rating Scale which can be used for clinical assessment

Table 6

FAD Criteria

	Family Assessmet Device (FAD)
Theoretical Domain and Model	Family System McMaster Model
Assessment Level	Family as Whole
Number of Scales and Items	7 Scales; 53 Items
Norms	
Normative Sample	n = 503 Adults
Clinical	Variety of Clinical Samples in Progress
Reliability	
Internal Consistency	Very good evidence
Test-Retest	X = .71
Validity	
Face Validity	Very good evidence
Content Validity	Very good evidence
Correlation Between Scales	X = .56
Correlation with Social Desirability	Range = −.06 to .19 (n = 164)
Concurrent Validity	Good evidence
Correlation Between Family Members	Lack of Evidence
Discrimination Between Groups	Good evidence
Clinical Utility	
Usefulness of Self-report Scale	Very good evidence
Ease of Administering and Scoring	Good evidence, but no existing manual
Clinical Rating Scale	Yes
Ethnic Diversity Utility	Some evidence

of families and for obtaining ratings from therapists. A recent study (Fristad, 1989) found that every scale except for Affective Responsiveness had significant correlations (.39 to .69) between the FAD and its clinical rating scale. There is some indication that a few of the clinical scales may be hard to score, and the choice of words on some items may be problematic (Fristad, 1989).

In terms of application to ethnic diversity issues, the FAD was recently used with Hawaiian-American and Japanese-American groups in conjunction with a structured interview (Morris, 1990). Results indicated that, when FAD scores were compared to the interviews, the FAD had incorrectly assessed the Japanese-Americans with regard to affective responses and behavior control. Compared to the FAD norms, the Japanese-American group scored in the emotionally constricted range with a rigid style of behavior. However, this was not consistent with the interview data. It is possible the self-report data reflects the traditional views and values of Japanese-Americans (Table 6).

3. FAMILY ASSESSMENT MEASURE (FAM III)

Theoretical Domain

The Family Assessment Measure (FAM III) is built on the Process Model of Family Functioning which attempts to integrate various perspectives of family therapy and research (Steinhauer et al., 1984). The Process Model builds on the Family Categories Schema developed by Epstein, Baldwin, and Bishop (1981) in that similar dimensions of family behavior were identified as important for understanding family functioning.

The specific variables in the Process Model include task accomplishment, role performance, communication, affective expression, involvement, control, and values and norms. Definitions of these scales are presented in the Table (Table 7).

While the FAM focuses on the family system, it also provides an assessment of dyadic functioning. The most recent version of the instrument is FAM III. It consists of three components: A *General Scale* which focuses on the family as a system; a *Dyadic Relationship Scale* which examines relationships between specific pairs in the family; and a *Self-Rating Scale* which taps the individual's perception of his or her functioning in the family (Skinner et al., 1983). Each of these major scales assesses the seven important dimensions of family functioning, but each provides a different perspective on how the family system operates. The Dyadic Scale appears to be much more sensitive to dysfunction than the General Scale.

The FAM III consists of three specific assessment components—the General Scale consisting of 50 items, the Dyadic Scale consisting of 42 items, and the Self-Rating Scale consisting of 42 items. The General Scale also includes two response style measures: social desirability (seven items) and defensiveness (eight items). If all three scales are used, there is a minimum total of 134 items, depending upon how many dyadic units

TABLE 7: FAMILY ASSESSMENT MEASURE (FAM II)

Affective Involvement	This is the degree and quality of family member's interest and concern for one another. This will determine whether the relationships are nurturing and supportive or destructive and self-serving. There are five types of family affective involvement: (1) uninvolved, (2) interest and devoid of feeling, (3) narcissistic, (4) empathic and (5) enmeshed.
Control	This described a variety of interpersonal strategies or techniques used to influence another member's behavior. There are four types of family control: (1) rigid, (2) flexible, (3) laissez-faire and (4) chaotic.
Role Performance	Roles are prescribed in repetitive behaviors involving a set of reciprocal activities with other family members. These roles either facilitate or impede successful task accomplishment. Roles can be classified into either traditional or idiosyncratic.
Task Accomplishment	This is the central focus of the process model. While some of the family tasks are culturally defined, others are defined by the family's norms and values. There are basically three types of tasks: (1) basic tasks, (2) developmental tasks and (3) crises tasks.
Communication	This is a mechanism through which formation for affective role performance and task accomplishment is exchanged. The content of communication can be affective, instrumental or neutral.
Affective Expression	This is a vital element in effective communication. It includes the content, intensity and timing of feelings expressed and it is the most often distorted in times of stress.
Values and Norms	These provide the background against which all basic processes must be considered. It includes whether family rules are explicit or implicit, the latitude for members to determine their own attitudes, and whether family norms are consistent with the broader cultural context.

within the family are assessed. Most current users of FAM III incorporate all three scales.

Reliability and Validity

The norms for FAM III are based on 312 individuals (Skinner et al., 1984). Some norms have also been developed with an extensive sample of clinical families. To date, there is a total of 53 published studies using FAM.

The internal consistency reliability of the three scales is excellent: .93 for the General Scale, .95 for the Dyadic Relationship Scale, and .89 for the Self-Rating Scale. The reliability for the subscales within each of these major scales is somewhat lower but still acceptable. The median reliability for the nine subscales in the General Scale was .73; for the six subscales in the Dyadic Relationship Scale it was .72; and for the six subscales in the Self-Rating Scale the median reliability was .53.

At this time there is a lack of evidence on the test-retest reliability of any of these three primary scales.

In terms of concurrent validity, there is a lack of evidence on the correlation of these scales with other approaches to family assessment. However, both face and content validity for all three scales appear adequate.

One of the somewhat problematic issues for these three primary scales is that there appears to be a strong general factor of family functioning. This is revealed by the rather high intercorrelations among the subscales of each of the major scales. Skinner (1987) found the following correlations between the subscales: General Scale, .39 to .70; Dyadic Relationship Scale, .68 to .82; Self-Rating Scale, .25 to .63.

Another somewhat problematic issue is the correlation of social desirability with each of the scales: General Scale = −.53, Dyadic Scale = −.35, and Self-Rating Scale = −.35.

The correlation between family members' responses on the General Scale was .36 for normal couples and .51 for clinical couples. This level of correlation between family members is typical of what has been found in other studies of family functioning that use self-report methods (Olson et al., 1983).

The ability of FAM III to discriminate between problem families and non-problem families was examined in a recent study by Skinner et al. (1987). Families who had a member receiving professional/clinical help were more likely to score poorly on role performance and involvement subscales than non-problem families. Recently, a study of 76 families who had a child with school phobia were assessed (Bernstein et al., 1990). The parent-child dyad was rated dysfunctional in the areas of role performance and values and norms. Westhues and Cohen (1990) examined families in which special-needs adoptions were successful versus disrupted. A discriminant function analysis showed the FAM was able to correctly predict between the two groups in over 90% of the cases, based largely on the wife's values and norms and the husband's involvement.

Clinical Utility

The FAM III takes about 30-45 minutes to administer. It may be completed by family members as young as 10-12 years of age. Testing materials must be obtained by the project coordinator, and plans are underway to have FAM III formally published within the year.

Goals for developing this inventory were not only to assess both individual intrapsychic functioning and total family system functioning, but also to provide data that are clinically useful (Steinhauer, 1984; Steinhauer & Tisdall, 1984). The clinical usefulness of this model appears promising. Some caution has been expressed as to FAM III's sensitivity to detect changes in family functioning as measured before and after a clinical treatment program (Blackman et al., 1986). A structured interview and clinical rating scale are currently still being tested.

No information is available about the FAM III's utility for ethnically diverse samples (Table 8).

4. FAMILY ENVIRONMENT SCALE (FES)

Theoretical Domain

The Family Environment Scale (FES) was one of the earliest self-report assessment scales developed; it was based on dimensions which were found useful in studying the social climate of families (Moos, 1974). The criteria for evaluating the FES and a summary of this evaluation are provided in Table 10.

The FES contains ten scales which are divided into three major dimensions. The conceptual definitions of these ten scales are provided in Table 9.

The *Relationship Dimension* consists of the three scales of cohesion, expressiveness, and conflict. The *Personal Growth Dimension* consists of

Table 8

FAM III Criteria

	Family Assessment Measure (FAM III)
Theoretical Domain and Model	Family System Process Model
Assessment Level	Family, Dyadic and Individual
Number of Scales and Items	General Scale (50 items) Dyadic (42 items) Self-Rating (42 items)

Norms
  Normative Sample
  Clinical
	
	Norms Based on 312 Individuals
	Variety of Clinical Families

Reliability
  Internal Consistency
 	
  Test-Retest
	
	Excellent evidence
	General Scale (r = .93)
	Dyadic (r = .95)
	Self-Rating Scale (r = .89)
	Lack of Evidence

Validity
  Face Validity
  Content Validity
  Correlation between Scales
  Correlation with Social Desirability
 	
  Concurrent Validity
  Correlation Between Family
  Members
 	
  Discrimination Between Groups
	
	Very good evidence
	Very good evidence
	X = .25 to .82
	r = −.53 General Scale & SD
	r = −.35 Dyadic Scale & SD
	r = −.35 Self-Rating & SD
	Lack of evidence
	
	H/W on General Scale
	r = .36 Normal Couples
	r = .51 Clinical Couples
	Good evidence

Clinical Utility
  Usefulness of Self-report Scale
  Ease of Administering and Scoring
  Clinical Rating Scale
  Ethnic Diversity Utility
	
	Very good evidence
	Very easy
	Not yet published
	Lack of evidence

TABLE 9: FAMILY ENVIRONMENT SCALE (FES)

Relationship Dimensions	
Cohesion	Commitment, help and support family members provide for one another.
Expressiveness	How much family members are encouraged to act openly and to express their feelings directly.
Conflict	The amount of openly expressed anger, aggression and conflict among family members.
Personal Growth Dimension	
Independence	The extent to which family members are assertive, self-sufficient, and make their own decisions.
Achievement Orientation	The extent to which activities (e.g., school and work) are cast into an achievement-oriented or competitive framework.
Intellectual-Cultural Orientation	The degree of interest in political, social, intellectual and cultural activities.
Active-Recreational Orientation	Extent of participation in social and recreational activities.
Moral-Religious Emphasis	Emphasis on ethical and religious issues and values.
System Maintenance Dimensions	
Organization	The importance of clear organization and structure in planning family activities and responsibilities.
Control	Extent to which set rules and procedures are used to run family life.

five scales: independence, achievement orientation, intellectual-cultural orientation, active-recreational orientation, and moral-religious emphasis. The *System Maintenance Dimension* consists of the two scales of organization and control. There are nine items for each of the ten scales.

The assessment level of FES is on the family as a whole. The focus of the assessment can be on current family functioning (real form), ideal family functioning (ideal form), and an individual's expectations about family functioning (expectation form). Each of these separate forms consists of a 90-item, true-false questionnaire (Table 9).

While the initial study for developing norms for the FES was based on a sample of 285 families (Moos, 1974), an updated manual (Moos & Moos, 1986, 2nd ed.) describes the updated norms based on 1,428 adults and 621 adolescents. The final normal sample consists of 1,125 families, and norms for 500 distressed families.

Reliability and Validity

In terms of reliability, the internal consistency reliability of ten scales was good. The average reliability was .73, the range was .61 to .78. The test-retest reliability also was good, ranging from .68 to .86 for eight weeks, and from .52 to .89 for one year.

In terms of face validity, the items do appear to measure what they were intended to measure. For content validity, there seems to be a good representative range of relevant issues for each of these scales.

Construct validity has been examined by several investigators, resulting in some inconsistent findings. Fowler (1981, 1982) conducted a factor analysis which revealed two major factors: (1) cohesion versus conflict, and (2) organization and control. This supports some of the earlier theoretical work (Olson et al., 1983) which emphasizes the salience of the two dimensions of cohesion and adaptability. In a factor analysis by Robertson and Hyde (1982), seven areas were identified instead of the ten which comprise the subscales. Although Nelson (1984) identified three factors in his study of middle-school aged children, they differed from the original three dimensions described by Moos.

When correlations between the ten scales are reviewed, there appears to be a moderate level of correlation between the scales. Fowler (1982) indicated the correlation of the scales with social desirability ranged from .02 for moral-religious emphasis to .44 for cohesion. A study of 183 undergraduates by Schmid et al. (1988) using two FES scales (cohesion and control) found correlations with social desirability of .10 and .01, respectively.

Concurrent validity of the FES is somewhat mixed. At least two different modified multi-trait multi-method analyses have revealed different results. One by Russell (1980) found the FES cohesion scale did not correlate with the other three self-report or behavioral assessments of cohesion. Another analysis by Schmid and others (1988) showed FES cohesion correlated with FACES II cohesion .74, while FES control correlated −.32

with FACES adaptability. On the other hand, Oliveri and Reiss (1984) found no significant correlations between Reiss' Card Sort procedure and the FES.

In terms of discriminant validity, more than 200 studies have demonstrated that the FES discriminates between different types of families. One approach has been the use of cluster analysis in which 100 families were clustered into six family types (Moos & Moos, 1976). The FES also has been found to be very useful in discriminating distressed families (Moos & Moos, 1981) and indicating changes as a result of alcoholism treatment (Finney et al., 1980, 1983; Moos & Moos, 1984; Moos et al., 1979, 1981, 1982).

More recently, Dinning and Berk (1989) found differences among a sample of children of alcoholics. Those who indicated more distress with a parent's drinking scored lower in family cohesion and overall family support, and higher in family conflict. A study about stepfamilies (Brown et al., 1990) distinguished between those in therapy for a child-focused problem and those not in therapy, with no child-focused problems. The latter group reported higher expressiveness and lower conflict than the therapy group.

Clinical Utility

The clinical utility of the FES scale appears to be quite good. Fuhr, Moos, and Dishotsky (1981) compared a family's real description (Form R) and ideal description (Form I) of the family environment to identify areas needing change. Moos and Fuhr (1982) also illustrated how FES can be used to complete a clinical assessment and formulate intervention strategies.

The FES is rather easy to administer and score. The possibility of using the various 90-item forms becomes problematic in major outcome studies because of the length of each form (n = 90 items). However, a modified version of the FES has recently been used as a measure of family environment. The Family Relationship Index (FRI) is a composite of the family cohesion, expressiveness, and conflict subscales of the FES, and has only 27 items. Hoge and others (1989) investigated the construct validity of the FRI by comparing scores of families in counseling to evaluations by family therapists. Correlations between the FRI and therapists' ratings ranged from −.27 to −.46. At the present time there is no clinical rating scale for the FES.

The sample from which the FES was normed reportedly included diverse family characteristics. Baranowski and others (1986) examined the psychometric properties of the FES with Anglo, African-American and Mexican-American adult family members. Internal consistency was rather low, although showed highest for the Anglo sample, and the factor analysis revealed subscales within the original dimensions. The authors suggest that reading abilities, inappropriate items, and lack of real-life relevance to the other two ethnic groups may have contributed to the results.

Munet-Vilaro and Egan (1990) used the FES in two different cross-cultural studies, with Puerto Rican families and Vietnamese foster families. Internal consistency reliability was not strong, but contributing factors may have been due to translation inadequacies, dissimilar values, or use of colloquialism (Table 10).

5. SELF-REPORT FAMILY INVENTORY (SFI)

Theoretical Domain

The Self-report Family Inventory (SFI) is based on the Beavers Systems Model of Family Functioning (BSM), which derives from three main sources: general systems theory, clinical work with families, and research.

The SFI contains six scales which are designed to measure family members' perceptions of their family's health, conflict, communication, cohesion, directive leadership, and expressiveness. The conceptual definitions are provided in Table 11. A second order factor analysis has collapsed the previous six areas into (a) health/competence, (b) style, and (c) expressiveness. These three factors are reportedly congruent with the observational instruments of the BSM (Table 11).

Reliability and Validity

The norms for the SFI are based on 186 families (Grotevant & Cooper, 1989). Reliability characteristics show very good internal consistency, assessed at between .84 and .88. The test-retest reliability was assessed at 30 and 90 days, and was strongest for family health and expressiveness scales. Test-retest reliability was not strong for the scales of communication (.39) and directive leadership (.44).

Face validity of the scales appears very good. Content validity might be of concern for those

Table 10

FES Criteria

	Family Environment Scale (FES)
Theoretical Domain and Model	Family Climate Social Psychological Model
Assessment Level	Family as Whole
Focus of Assessment	Real; Ideal; Expectation
Number of Scales and Items	10 Scales; 90 Items
Norms	
Normative Sample	n = 1,498 Adults
	n = 621 Adolescents
Clinical	n = 500 Distressed Families
Reliability	
Internal Consistency	Good evidence; X = .73; Range = .61 to .78
Test-Retest	.68 to .86 for 8 weeks; .52 to .8 for one year
Validity	
Face Validity	Very good evidence
Content Validity	Very good evidence
Correlation Between Scales	X = .20
Correlation with Social Desirability	Range = .02 to .44
Concurrent Validity	Mixed
Correlation Between Family	
Members	Lack of Evidence
Discrimination Between Groups	Very good evidence
Clinical Utility	
Usefulness of Self-report Scale	Very good evidence
Ease of Administering and Scoring	Good evidence
Clinical Rating Scale	Not developed
Ethnic Diversity Utility	Some evidence

TABLE 11: SELF-REPORT FAMILY INVENTORY (SFI)

Overall Competence Dimension	
Family Health/Competence Factor	Items involving happiness, optimism, problem-solving abilities, parental coalitions, allowance for individuality, acceptance of individuals and love in the home, low blaming behaviors.
Behavioral & Emotional Style Dimensions	
Conflict	Items concerning fighting, arguing, blaming, problem-solving vs. unresolved conflict, acceptance of personal responsibility, and negative feeling tone in the family.
Communication	Items involving direct, open discussions, speaking one's mind directly, and open conflict resolution.
Cohesion	Items concerning togetherness, satisfaction derived from inside the family vs. outside, and spending time together.
Directive Leadership	Parental leadership and directive leadership vs. rigid control in the family.
Positive Emotional Expression	Open expression of warmth, caring and closeness, by verbal or nonverbal means.

scales which consist of four items or less (family communication and directive leadership). Correctional analysis between the scales was not reported. None of the correlations between social desirability and each scale was significant.

In terms of concurrent validity, the SFI has been extensively tested. SFI scales have for the most part shown moderate to strong correlations with other scales (e.g., FACES II and III, Bloom Family Evaluation Scale, FES, and FAD). The "health" scale shows the strongest correlation with other measures, while the communication scale has yielded inconsistent results.

There is evidence that the dimensions of health/competence and expressiveness were able to discriminate between high and low functioning families. In one pilot study, emergency room psychiatric patients were diagnosed by hospital staff while accompanying family members completed the SFI. Initial results show a relationship between Beaver's Model of family style and psychiatric disorder (Beavers & Hampson, 1990).

Clinical Utility

The SRI was initially designed to be used in conjunction with the observational ratings scales of the Beavers Systems Model of Family Functioning, and the clinical utility appears quite good. No special training procedures are necessary, although a familiarization with the Beavers Systems Model is helpful. The manual includes scoring and psychometric information.

There are two observational rating scales: the Beavers-Timberlawn Family Evaluation Scale (Lewis, Beavers, Gossett, & Phillips, 1976) and the Centripetal/Centrifugal Family Style Scale

(Kelsey-Smith & Beavers, 1981). The former assesses family competence, while the latter measures family style.

With regard to ethnic diversity issues, more results are reported for the observational rating scales than for the SFI. Studies of European-American, African-American and Mexican-American families have found no differences in competence or style, but some observed differences in interaction patterns (Beavers & Hampson, 1990). The criteria for evaluating the SFI are reported in the Table (Table 12).

CONCLUSIONS

Table 13 provides an indicator of concurrent validity among four of the scales. The five self-report inventories of family functioning selected for this review represent the state of the art. All five inventories are derived from a theoretical framework and each of these instruments has been studied in terms of reliability, validity and clinical utility. For each of these inventories, there is a commitment to continually improve their scientific rigor and clinical usefulness, including their application to diverse ethnic samples. Also, all of these inventories are being used currently in ongoing research (Table 13).

Although the self-report instrument may be the most widely used research tool, the assessment of family functioning is far from finalized. It is our hope that professionals in the family field will continue to further their cooperative efforts to bridge research, theory and practice, to the benefit of each and the advancement of family science.

Table 12

SFI Criteria

	Self-report Family Inventory (SFI)
Theoretical Domain and Model	Family Systems Beavers Systems Model of Family Functioning
Assessment Level	Family as Whole
Focus of Assessment	Perceived Real
Number of Scales and Items	6 Scales; 36 Items
Norms	N = 186 Families (Grotevant)
Reliability	
Internal Consistency	Very good; Range = .84 to .88
Test-Retest	X = .60
Validity	
Face Validity	Very good evidence
Content Validity	Good evidence
Correlation Between Scales	Lack of evidence
Correlation with Social Desirability	Range = –.03 to .11
Concurrent Validity	Very good evidence
Correlation Between Family Members	Pilot studies range from .11 to .67
Discrimination Between Groups	Very good evidence
Clinical Utility	
Usefulness of Self-report Scale	Very good evidence
Ease of Administering and Scoring	Very good evidence
Clinical Rating Scale	Two: Beavers-Timberlawn Family Evaluation Scale Centripetal/Centrifugal Family Style Scale
Ethnic Applicability	Some evidence for SFI

Table 13

Correlations Between SFI and 3 Family Instruments

FES*

SFI	Cohesion	Expressive-ness	Conflict	Independence	Achieve-ment	Intellectual-Cultural Orientation	Active-Recreational Orientation	Moral-Religious Emphasis	Organization	Control
Family health	-.73	-.50	.66	.26	.14 (n.s.)	-.40	-.38	-.21	-.18 (n.s.)	.28
Conflict	-.48	-.35	-.68	-.19 (n.s.)	.29	-.13	-.18 (n.s.)	-.23	-.25	.17 (n.s.)
Family communication	-.16 (n.s.)	-.40	.23	-.21	-.14 (n.s.)	-.10 (n.s.)	-.06 (n.s.)	.03 (n.s.)	.04 (n.s.)	.37
Family cohesion	-.65	-.37	.49	-.24	.14 (n.s.)	-.32	-.23	-.09 (n.s.)	-.14 (n.s.)	.22
Directive leadership	-.24	.10 (n.s.)	.17 (n.s.)	-.09 (n.s.)	-.19 (n.s.)	-.25	-.01 (n.s.)	-.31	-.24	-.38
Expressiveness	-.71	-.39	.59	-.05 (n.s.)	.97 (n.s.)	-.35	-.22	-.22	-.16 (n.s.)	.21

N = 71

*Beavers and Hampson, 1990

n.s. = not significant

Table 13 (continued)

SFI	Problem Solving	Communication	Roles	Affective Responsiveness	Affective Involvement	Behavior Control	General Functioning
				FAD*			
Family health	.55	.58	.47	.64	.54	.08 (n.s.)	.77
Conflict	.29	.38	.33	.41	.53	.14 (n.s.)	.53
Family communication	.20 (n.s.)	.35	.11 (n.s.)	.07 (n.s.)	.24	–.21	.27
Family cohesion	.45	.57	.29	.61	.30	–.11 (n.s.)	.61
Directive leadership	.27	.18 (n.s.)	.34	.13 (n.s.)	.29	.36	.27
Expressiveness	.62	.63	.48	.69	.43	.12 (n.s.)	.68

N = 71

*Beavers and Hampson, 1990

n.s. = not significant

94

Table 13 (continued)

SFI	FACES**					
	Adaptability		Cohesion			
	II	III		II	III	
Family health	-.79	-.22		-.93	-.78	
Conflict	-.55	.02 (n.s.)		-.69	-.45	
Family communication	-.30	-.17 (n.s.)		-.12 (n.s.)	-.18 (n.s.)	
Family cohesion	-.59	-.17 (n.s.)		-.81	-.67	
Directive leadership	-.49	-.39		-.62	-.37	
Expressiveness	-.35	-.18 (n.s.)		-.58	-.73	

II - N = 279
III - N = 71

**Hampson, Hulgus, and Beavers, 1990

n.s. = not significant

REFERENCES

Barnes, H. L., & Olson, D. H. (1982). Parent-adolescent communication scale. In D. H. Olson, H. I. McCubbin, H. Barnes, A. Larsen, M. Muxen, & M. Wilson (Eds.), *Family Inventories*, (pp. 51-66). St. Paul, MN: University of Minnesota, Family Social Science.

Barnes, H. L., & Olson, D. H. (1985). Parent adolescent communication and the circumplex model. *Child Development, 56*, 438-447.

Baranowski, T., Dworkin, R. J., Hooks, P., Nader, P. R., & Brown J. (1986). The reliability of two measures of family functioning in three ethnic groups. *Family Perspective, 20*(4):353-364.

Beavers, W. R., & Hampson, R. B. (1990). *Successful families: Assessment and intervention,* (p. 237). New York: W.W. Norton.

Bernstein, G. A., Svingen, P. H., & Garfinkel, B. D. (1990). School phobia: Patterns of family functioning. *Journal of the American Academy Child Adolescent Psychiatry, 29*(1):24-39.

Bishop, D. S., & Epstein, N. B. (1985). Training family physicians to treat families: Response to Hochheiser and Chapados. *Family Systems Medicine, 3*(4): 481-485.

Bishop, D. S., & Epstein, N. B. (1987). Family therapy and the family physician: Where to family medicine, where to family training. *Family Systems Medicine, 5*(3).

Blackman, M., Pitcher, S., & Rauch, F. (1986). A preliminary outcome study of a community group treatment program for emotionally disturbed adolescents. *Canadian Journal of Psychiatry, 31*:112-118.

Brown, A. C., Green, R. J., Druckman, J. (1990). A comparison of stepfamilies with and without child-focused problems. *American Journal of Orthopsychiatry, 60*(4):556-566.

Byles, J., Byrne, C., Boyle, M., & Offord, D. (1988). Ontario child health study: Reliability and validity of the general functioning subscale of the McMaster Family Assessment Device. *Family Process, 27*: 97-104.

Campbell, D. T., & Fiske, D. W. (1959). Convergent and discriminant validation by the multitrait-multimethod matrix. *Psychological Bulletin, 56*:81-105.

Dinning, W. D., & Berk, L. A. The children of alcoholics screening test: Relationship to sex, family environment, and social adjustment in adolescents. *Journal of Clinical Psychology, 45*(2):335-339.

Epstein, N. B., Baldwin, L., & Bishop, D. (1983). The McMaster Family Assessment Device. *Journal of Marital & Family Therapy, 9*(2):213-228.

Epstein, N. B., & Bishop, D. (1981). Problem centered systems therapy of the family. *Journal of Marital & Family Therapy, 7*, 23-31.

Epstein, N. B., Baldwin, L., & Bishop, D. S. (1981). McMaster Model of family functioning: A view of the normal family. In F. Walsh (Ed.), *Normal Family Processes.* New York, NY: Guilford.

Epstein, N. B., Keitner, G. E., Bishop, D. S., & Miller, I. W. (1988). Clinical experiences with a combination of pharmacological and family Rx of the affective disorders. In J. Clarkin, G. Haas, & I. Glick (Eds.), *Family variables and interventions in affective illness.* New York, NY: Guilford.

Epstein, N. B., Sigal, J., & Rakoff, V. (1968). *Family categories schema.* Unpublished manuscript, Jewish General Hospital, Montreal, Canada.

Finney, J. W., Moos, R. H., Cronkite, R. C., & Gamble, W. (1980). A conceptual model of the functioning of married persons with impaired partners: Spouses of alcoholic patients. *Journal of Marriage & the Family, 45*, 23-34.

Finney, J. W., Moos, R. H., & Newborn, C. R. (1980). Post-treatment experiences and treatment outcome of alcoholic patients six months and two years after hospitalization. *Journal of Consulting and Clinical Psychology, 48*:17-29.

Fowler, P. C. (1981). Maximum likelihood factor structure of the Family Environment Scale. *Journal of Clinical Psychology, 37*, 160-164.

Fowler, P. C. (1982). Factor structure of the Family Environment Scale: Effects of social desirability. *Journal of Clinical Psychology, 38*, 285-292.

Fredman, N., & Sherman, R. (1987). *Handbook of measurements of marriage and family therapy,* (pp. 218). New York, NY: Brunner/Mazel.

Fristad, M. A. (1989). A comparison of the McMaster and Circumplex family assessment instruments. *Journal of Marital & Family Therapy, 15*(3): 259-269.

Fuhr, R. A., Moos, R. H., & Dishotsky, N. (1981). The use of family assessment and feedback in ongoing family therapy. *American Journal of Family Therapy, 9*, 24-36.

Green, R. G. (1989). Choosing family measurement devices for practice and research: SFI and FACES III. *Social Science Review, 63*, 304-320.

Grotevant, H. D., & Carlson, C. I. (1989). *Family assessment: A guide to methods and measures,* (pp. 500). New York, NY: Guilford Press.

Hampson, R. B., Hulgus, Y. F., & Beavers, W. R. (1991). Comparisons of self-report measures of the Beavers Systems Model and Olson's Circumplex Model. *Journal of Family Psychology, 4*(3):326-340.

Hoge, R. A., Andrews, D. A., Faulkner, P., & Robinson, D. (1989). The family relationship index: Validity data. *Journal of Clinical Psychology, 45*(6):897-903.

Hulgus, Y. F., Hampson, R. B., & Beavers, W. R. (1985). *Self-report family inventory.* Dallas, TX: Southwest Family Institute.

Jacob, T., & Tennenbaum, D. L. (1988). *Family assessment: Rationale, methods, and future directions,* (pp. 208). New York, NY: Plenum.

Kabacoff, R. I., Miller, I. W., Bishop, D. S., Epstein, N. B., & Keitner, G. I. (1990). A psychometric study of the McMaster Family Assessment Device in psychiatric, medical and nonclinical samples. *Journal of Family Psychology, 3*(4):431-439.

Keitner, G. I., (Ed.). (1990). *Depression and families: Impact on treatment.* Washington, DC: American Psychiatric Press.

Kelsey-Smith, M., & Beavers, W. R. Family assessment: Centripetal and centrifugal family systems. *American Journal of Family Therapy, 9*, 3-21.

Lewis, J. M., Beavers, W. R., Gossett, J. T., & Phillips, V. A. (1976). *No single thread: Psychological health in family systems.* New York, NY: Brunner/Mazel.

Markman, H. J., & Notarius, C. I. (1987). Coding marital and family interaction: Current status. In T. J.

96

Jacob, (Ed.). *Family Interaction and Psychopathology.* New York, NY: Plenum.

Miller, I. W., Epstein, N. B., Bishop, D. S., & Keitner, G. I. (1985). The McMaster Family Assessment Device: Reliability and validity. *Journal of Marital & Family Therapy, 11*(4):345-356.

Moos, R. (1974). *Combined preliminary manual for the family, work, and group environment scales.* Palo Alto, CA: Consulting Psychologists Press.

Moos, R., Bromet, E., Tsu, V., & Moos, B. (1979). Family characteristics and the outcome of treatment for alcoholism. *Journal of Studies on Alcohol, 40,* 78-88.

Moos, R., Finney, J., & Chan, D. A. (1981). The process of recovery from alcoholism: I. Comparing alcoholic patients and matched community controls. *Journal of Studies on Alcohol, 42,* 383-402.

Moos, R., Finney, J., & Gamble, W. (1982). The process of recovery from alcoholism: II. Comparing alcoholic patients and matched community controls. *Journal on Studies of Alcohol, 43,* 888-909.

Moos, R., & Fuhr, R. (1982). The clinical use of social-ecological concepts: The case of an adolescent girl. *American Journal of Orthopsychiatry, 52,* 111-112.

Moos, R., & Moos, B. (1976). A typology of family social environments. *Family Process, 15,* 357-372.

Moos, R., & Moos, B. (1981). *Family environment scale manual.* Palo Alto, CA: Consulting Psychologists Press.

Moos, R., & Moos, B. (1984). The process of recovery from alcoholism: III. Comparing functioning in families of alcoholics and matched control families. *Journal on Studies of Alcohol, 45,* 111-118.

Moos, R., & Moos, B. (1986). *Family environment scale manual* (2nd ed.). Palo Alto, CA: Consulting Psychologists Press.

Morris, T. M. (1990). Culturally sensitive family assessment: An evaluation of the Family Assessment Device used with Hawaiian-American and Japanese-American families. *Family Process, 29,* 105-116.

Munet-Vilaro, F., & Egan, M. (1990). Reliability issues of the Family Environment Scale for cross-cultural research. *Nursing Research, 39*(4):244-247.

Nelson, G. (1984). The relationship between dimensions of classroom and family environments and the self-concept, satisfaction, and achievement of grade 7 and 8 students. *Journal of Community Psychology, 12,* 276-287.

Oliveri, M. E., & Reiss, D. (1984). Family concepts and their measurement: Things are seldom what they seem. *Family Process, 23,* 33-48.

Olson, D. H. (1976). Bridging research, theory, and application: The triple threat in science. In D. H. Olson (Ed.), *Treating relationships,* (pp. 565-577). Lake Mills, IA: Graphic.

Olson, D. H. (1977). Insiders' and outsiders' views of relationships: Research studies. In G. Levinger & H. L. Raush (Eds.), *Close relationships: Perspectives on the meaning of intimacy,* (pp. 115-135). Amherst, MA: University of Massachusetts Press.

Olson, D. H. (1989). Circumplex Model and family health. In C. M. Ramsey (Ed.), *Family Systems Medicine,* (pp. 75-94). New York, NY: Guilford.

Olson, D. H. (1991). Commentary: Three-dimensional (3-D) circumplex model and revised scoring of FACES III. *Family Process, 30,* 74-79.

Olson, D. H., Fournier, D. G., & Druckman, J. M. (1982). *ENRICH: Evaluating and nurturing relationship issues, communication, happiness.* Minneapolis, MN: PREPARE/ENRICH, Inc.

Olson, D. H., McCubbin, H. I., Barnes, H. L., Larsen, A. S., Muxen, M. J., & Wilson, M. A. (1989). *Families: What makes them work,* (pp. 310). Updated ed. Newbury Park, CA: Sage.

Olson, D. H., Portner, J., & Bell, R. Q. (1982). *FACES II: Family adaptability and cohesion evaluation scales.* St. Paul, MN: University of Minnesota, Family Social Science.

Olson, D. H., Portner, J., & Lavee, Y. (1985). *FACES III: Family adaptability and cohesion evaluation scales.* St. Paul, MN: University of Minnesota, Family Social Science.

Olson, D. H., Russell, C. S., & Sprenkle, D. H. (1980). Circumplex model of marital and family systems II: Empirical studies and clinical intervention. In J. Vincent (Ed.), *Advances in family intervention, assessment and theory* (Vol. I), (pp. 129-179). Greenwich, CT: JAI.

Olson, D. H., Russell, C. S., & Sprenkle, D. H. (1983). Circumplex Model of marital and family systems VI: Theoretical update. *Family Process, 22,* 69-83.

Olson, D. H., Sprenkle, D. H., & Russell, C. S. (1979). Circumplex Model of marital and family systems I: Cohesion and adaptability dimensions, family types, and clinical applications. *Family Process, 18,* 3-28.

Robertson, D. U., & Hyde, J. S. (1982). The factorial validity of the Family Environment Scale. *Educational Psychological Measurement, 42,* 1233-1241.

Russell, C. S. (1980). A methodological study of family cohesion and adaptability. *Journal of Marital & Family Therapy, 6,* 459-470.

Schmid, K. D., Rosenthal, S. L., & Brown, E. D. Comparison of self-report measures of two family dimensions: Control and cohesion. *American Journal of Family Therapy, 16,* 73-77.

Skinner, H. A. (1987). Self-report instruments for family assessment. In T. J. Jacob, (Ed.), *Family Interaction and Psychopathology,* (pp. 427-452). New York, NY: Plenum.

Skinner, H. A., Steinhauer, P. D., & Santa-Barbara, J. (1983). The family assessment measure. *Canadian Journal of Community Mental Health, 2*(2):91-105.

Skinner, H. A., Steinhauer, P. D., & Santa-Barbara, J. (1984). *The family assessment measure: Administration and interpretation guide.* Toronto, Ontario: Addiction Research Foundation.

Steinhauer, P. D. (1984). Clinical applications of the process model of family functioning. *Canadian Journal of Psychiatry, 29,* 98-111.

Steinhauer, P. D., Santa-Barbara, J., & Skinner, H. A. (1984). The process model of family functioning. *Canadian Journal of Psychiatry, 29,* 77-88.

Steinhauer, P. D., & Tisdall, G. W. (1984). The integrated use of individual and family psychotherapy. *Canadian Journal of Psychiatry, 29,* 89-97.

Thomas, V., & Olson, D. H. Problem families and the circumplex model: Observational assessment using the clinical rating scale (CRS). Submitted, 1991.

Touliatos, J., Perlmutter, B. F., & Straus, M. A. (Eds.). (1990). *Handbook of family measurement techniques*, (pp. 797). Newbury Park, CA: Sage.

Westhues, A., & Cohen, J. S. (1990). Preventing disruption of special-needs adoptions. *Child Welfare, 69*(2):141-155.

Westley, W. A., & Epstein, N. B. (1969). *The Silent Majority*. San Francisco: Jossey-Bass.

APPENDIX A: WHERE TO OBTAIN FAMILY INVENTORIES

Family Adaptability and Cohesion Evaluation Scales (FACES II or III)

David H. Olson, Ph.D., Director
Family Inventories Project
Department of Family Social Science
University of Minnesota
290 McNeal Hall
St. Paul, Minnesota 55108
612-625-7250

Family Assessment Device (FAD)

Ivan W. Miller, Ph.D., Director
Brown University Family Research Program
Butler Hospital
345 Blackstone Boulevard
Providence, Rhode Island 02906
401-455-6200

Family Assessment Measure (FAM III)

FAM Project Coordinator
Addiction Research Foundation
33 Russell Street
Toronto, Ontario M5S 2S1
416-595-6129

Family Environment Scale (FES)

Consulting Psychologists Press
577 College Avenue
Palo Alto, California 94306

Self-Report Family Inventory (SFI)

Southwest Family Institute
12532 Nuestra
Dallas, Texas 75230-1718
214-960-0550

WILLIAM J. DOHERTY, PH.D.
Professor, Family Social Science
University of Minnesota

Health and Family Interaction: What We Know

Of all the industrialized nations, the United States has had the most difficult time conceptualizing the role of family life in the health and illness of citizens. Perhaps because of the dominance of individualism in our country, we tend to split the individual from the family, just as we have tended to split the mind from the body. The traditional emphasis in health research and health policy has been on individual factors in health, illness, and health behavior, with the family context peripheral.

In the past two decades, however, there has been an increasing recognition among researchers and clinicians of the crucial role of family relationships and family interactions in health and illness. The two main factors in this increasing recognition appear to be the acknowledgment of the pivotal role of life style factors in health and the increased awareness of the family's role as a gatekeeper to the health care system. For example, studies indicate that smoking is learned first at home for many people, and that 7 illness episodes are treated at home for every one that is seen by a physician (Doherty & Campbell, 1988). The family is the hidden agent of health activity in the United States.

The purpose of this paper is to summarize the state of knowledge about the role of family interactions in health. I will use the Family Health and Illness Cycle (Figure 1) as a model to organize and categorize the large set of research findings in this area (Doherty & Campbell, 1988).

The model, which can best be read beginning with the "Two o'clock" position, represents both a family's experience with a health problem over time, and the major topic areas for families and health research. Note also that the arrows connecting each section of the model, The Health Care System, are intended to represent the importance of families' interactions with health professionals and the larger health care system. In each section of the paper, I will describe the current situation for family health data and highlight data needs.

FAMILY HEALTH PROMOTION AND DISEASE REDUCTION

Family interactions have been found to shape and maintain the major health behaviors that influence individual health: diet, exercise, cigarette smoking, and alcohol use. Family members develop common behavioral patterns that promote health or create risk in each of these behavioral domains (Baranowski et. al., 1982; Doherty & Campbell, 1988). Imagine a middle aged man who has never cooked for himself. His physician diagnoses him with hypertension and sends him home with a new diet, but does not attempt to win his wife's support for the dietary changes. Both research and clinical experience testify to the ineffectiveness of many health behavior interventions that do not take the family context into account (Campbell, 1986).

Despite a clear consensus about the role of family interactions in health promotion and disease prevention, there is relatively little accessible national data on the concordance of family health behaviors and how they relate to the health of family members. Data are either gathered at the

98

FIGURE 1. FAMILY HEALTH AND ILLNESS CYCLE

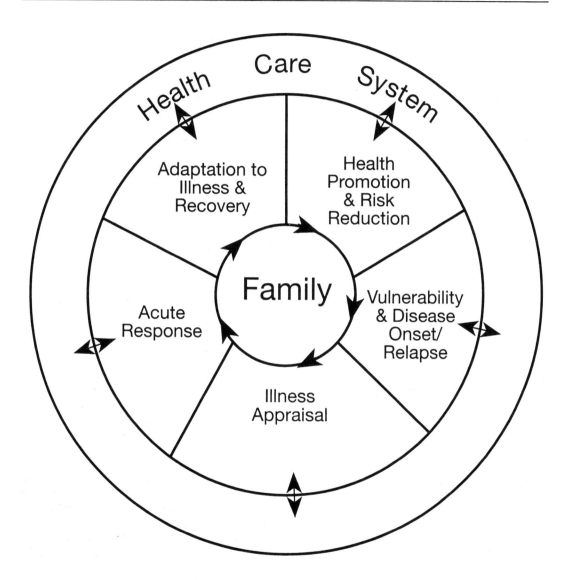

individual level, or are not easily analyzed at the family level when the household is the sampling unit. Needed are broad national surveys of the health behaviors of multiple family members.

FAMILY VULNERABILITY AND DISEASE ONSET/RELAPSE

Measures of stressful life events consistently rank family-related events, such as divorce and the death or serious illness of a family member, at the top of the list for creating distress. Recent studies, particularly in the field of psychoimmunology, have documented more specifically how family stress makes individuals vulnerable to illness. Widowers have been found to experience diminished immune system functioning following the death of their spouse (Calabrese et al., 1987). Divorced or separated individuals have poorer immune system functioning than matched married controls, and among married persons, those with poorer marital satisfaction have decreased immunity. Gottman and Katz (1989) have demonstrated a relationship between negative marital conflict and increased cortisol levels (a stress hormone) and poorer overall health among children. In sum, family stress is an important factor in creating susceptibility of illness among adults and children.

There is very little national data on how family stressful events and the quality of family relationships influence the health of individual family members. This is largely because national surveys tend to focus on individual symptoms and not on family contextual events and the quality of family bonds. Needed in surveys such as the National Health Interview Survey are items that inquire about family events such as divorce, that ask individuals to rate the quality of their marriages and other family relationships, and that simultaneously ask about individual health and illness.

FAMILY ILLNESS APPRAISAL

Family illness appraisal refers to the family's beliefs about illness and treatment. The family plays a pivotal role in assessing symptoms, encouraging home remedies, deciding whether professional help is needed, and gaining access to health care services (Doherty & Campbell, 1988). Families have broad beliefs, often based on cultural traditions, about how much they can control their destinies and how trustworthy professionals are (Reiss, 1981). They also have specific health beliefs related to symptoms and treatments, beliefs

which powerfully determine the individual's response to an illness episode (Gottlieb, 1976). Families' beliefs are the primary gateway to the health care system, as indicated by the finding that about seven illness episodes are treated at home for every one that is seen by a physician (Doherty & Campbell, 1988). Every family then, has its own epidemiology which it brings to its interactions with health professionals, and in many cases, the family's beliefs are more important in influencing outcomes than the formal diagnosis made by the health professional.

National surveys generally are deficient in inquiring about the health *beliefs* of individuals, focusing instead on health *behaviors* and health *problems*. Even more scarce are surveys that ask about multiple family members' beliefs. The result is often an emphasis on how to bring about health behavior changes without an appreciation for what certain practices mean to individuals and families. Needed are survey items inquiring about beliefs as well as behavior, and about multiple family members' beliefs as well as individuals' beliefs.

FAMILY ACUTE RESPONSE

As mentioned before, the onset of a serious illness in a family member is a highly stressful experience for both adults and children. This phase of the Family Health and Illness Cycle refers to the family's response in the short term aftermath of the onset of a serious illness episode. Research studies have shown that many families become temporarily overwhelmed but reorganize themselves to cope with the crisis; they call family members together and reach out to their social support network (Doherty & Campbell, 1988). Their greatest needs from the health care system are access to treatment and access to information. Coyne and Smith (1991), for example, found that a wife's distress, months after her husband's heart attack, was influenced by the adequacy of her initial contact with medical personnel during the acute response phase. Access and attention are the key issues for families during acute crises, along with the mobilization of their internal resources and social supports.

National surveys tell us relatively little about how families handle the acute response phase of their experience with serious illness. A payoff of gathering such data, even retrospectively, would be a greater understanding of how the trajectory is set during the acute phase for either good or poor family and individual adaptation during the chronic illness phase which often ensues.

FAMILY ADAPTATION TO ILLNESS OR RECOVERY

This is the largest area of research, families and health: how families deal with chronic illness and disability. Families during this phase often acquire a new role of caregiver for a family member—usually a wife or mother—along with a new role of "patient" for the ill members. This creates a set of imbalances for many families—between spouses, between parents and adult children, between siblings—that make chronic illness and disability a very challenging experience for many families (Doherty & Campbell, 1988). Studies indicate that the caregiver may be the most stressed member of the family, more so than the patient who is generally the object of clinical and research scrutiny (Oberst & James, 1985). Furthermore, families during this phase have ongoing and often stressful relationships with health care professionals and the health care system, relationships which can be seen as being as "chronic" as the illness (McDaniel, Hepworth, & Doherty, 1992). Not only does the illness affect the family, of course, but the quality of the lives of family members, especially the principal caregiver, is an important determinant of the health outcomes of ill family members (Campbell, 1986).

Along with family data on health behaviors, this area has the highest research priority, since so many families are providing the principal care for the chronically ill and disabled. It is important that national surveys give us more information about issues such as comorbidity among family members and the impact of a chronic illness on the emotional well-being of other family members. As the nation moves toward more in-home care, it is essential that we have good national data on the family connection to chronic illness and long term care.

In conclusion, family interactions are often the invisible thread interwoven into every aspect of health and health care. We need to know more about the intricacies of the dynamics of how families influence the health and illness of individuals, how the health and illness of individuals affect families, and how these forces are played out in the intricate patterning of family life. National surveys on broadly representative samples of families are a crucial ingredient in generating the knowledge needed to plan an effective, efficient, and caring health care system.

REFERENCES

Baranowski, T., Nader, P. R., Dunn, K., & Vanderpool, N. A. (1982, Summer). Family self-help: Promoting changes in health behavior. *Journal of Communication,* 161-172.

Calabrese, J. R., Kling, M. A., & Gold, P. W. (1987). Alterations in immunocompetence during stress, bereavement and depression: Focus on neuroendocrine regulation. *American Journal of Psychiatry, 144,* 1123-1134.

Campbell, T. L. (1986). *Family's impact on health: A critical review and annotated bibliography.* NIMH Series DN, No. 6. DHHS Publ. No (ADM) 86-1461. Also published in Family Systems Medicine, 1986, 4, 135-328.

Coyne, J. C., & Smith, D. A. F. (1991). Couples coping with a myocardial infarction: A contextual perspective on wives' distress. *Journal of Consulting and Clinical Psychology, 61,* 404-412.

Doherty, W. J., & Campbell, T. L. (1988). *Families and health.* Newbury Park, CA: Sage Publication.

Gottlieb, B. H. (1976). Lay influences on the utilization and provision of health services: A review. *Canadian Psychological Review, 17,* 126-136.

Gottman, J. M., & Katz, L. F. (1989). Effects of marital discord on young children's peer interaction and health. *Developmental Psychology, 25,* 373-381.

McDaniel, S. H., Hepworth, J. H., & Doherty, W. J. (1992). *Medical family therapy: A biopsychosocial approach to families with health problems.* New York: Basic Books.

Oberst, M. T., & James, R. H. (1985, April). Going home: Patient and spouse adjustment following cancer surgery. *Topics in Clinical Nursing,* 46-57.

Reiss, D. (1981). *The family's construction of reality.* Cambridge, MA: Harvard University Press.

THEODORA OOMS, M.S.W.
Director
Family Impact Seminar

Implications of Family Health and

Family Data on Policy

Ms. Ooms submitted a transcript of her presentation in lieu of a prepared paper.

Perhaps because I am a user of data rather than a researcher, I can stick my neck out and say that I think the issues being discussed at this conference represent the cutting edge of health care research and health care practice. They have profound implications for health care policy and health care reform. What do I mean by cutting edge? The recent Bill Moyers television series on the mind-body connection was a vivid and powerful statement in favor of the biopsychosocial paradigm of health and healing, which is a large part of what we are talking about here. Moyers made two essential points: one, that illness is clearly not solely a function of biological processes, and two, that healing is not the exclusive province of biomedical treatment. He made these points very well.

However, regrettably, he left out the fact that the most important psychosocial context is the family, and he paid scant attention to the role of the family in health and healing that the earlier panelists have outlined so thoroughly.

Another bit of evidence that you're on the cutting edge. I think we have all come to realize that if you shift from a focus on individuals to a focus on families in research or practice, it adds enormous complexity to data collection and analysis.

Just in case you sometimes get discouraged and feel it is not worth it, I would like to draw your attention to a marvelous book some of you may have come across, titled *Complexity* by Mitchell Waldrup. Its subtitle is *The Emerging Science at the Edge of Order and Chaos*. It is the story of the founding of the Sante Fe Institute in the 1980s by a group of mathematicians, physicists, computer scientists and economists who formed an iconoclastic think tank designed to create a new science called the science of complexity.

The fascination with complexity emerged as these scientists began to realize that a lot of nature was in fact not linear, including most of what is really interesting in the world. I think the ideas in this book have some relevance to what we are all doing in our work. Maybe we should set up our own Sante Fe think tank.

I will first comment briefly about the implications of the research we already have, as well as the research we would like to have for policy and practice. Second, mindful of the fact that money is tight and some of the items on our wish list for research may have to wait, I want to put forward a proposal which will be familiar to some of you of how we could go about improving the coordination and utilization of data that is already collected.

On both of these topics, I draw heavily on the collaborative work we have been involved with at the Family Impact Seminar with representatives of the five member Consortium of Family

Organizations, most notably the National Council on Family Relations, as well as my own parent organization, the Association for Marriage and Family Therapy.

Now, the implications of family data and family health on policy. I think it is safe to assume that the audience for the research conducted by most of you in this room is most immediately other researchers. But sooner or later, you expect and hope that the findings will be useful to health care practitioners and policy makers.

In our seminars we organize on Capitol Hill, we package and present the findings of surveys and research such as yours to help policy makers enact and implement policies that strengthen and support families in carrying out the various roles, particularly the health care role. We function as an intermediary, as a translator or broker, if you like, between those that produce data and research and the people in government. I think it is really important to underscore that busy policy makers and their staff have a terribly difficult time keeping up with all the information that is produced on families, and interpreting and understanding it, and then figuring out the implications for policy. The advocacy organizations have some of the same difficulty. They don't know where to go for information, and when they do get hold of it, they don't have time to read through it and sift what it means. So we really need to think a lot about how what you're learning can be translated into the policy arena.

Some of our seminars have focused on health issues. In the course of preparing these seminars, we have searched for information about family health status and all the issues that we have been talking about today. You will not be surprised to hear that all too often, the data we are looking for isn't there. It isn't collected at all, or it isn't tabulated in a way that is useful, or it is generally inaccessible, at least in the time we have to prepare.

But on the other hand, the question is, although we do need to know a great deal more, and it certainly needs to be more accessible, from what we know already, once the powerful role of the family in health care is understood, what is the bottom line for policy? Ron Haskins said that we need to give a simple message to the policy makers, even though the research may be very complicated, and it has to be a message that we can all agree to.

I believe the bottom line that has run through everything today is that family is very important in health and must not continue to be ignored. We don't understand all the combinations and processes and the ways in which families affect health. But the bottom line is that we must find more effective ways of involving family members as active partners in health care.

As we stated in the COFO health care reform white paper, which I think some of you have seen, the health care system needs to become more family centered and family friendly (COFO, 1992). This means changes at all levels of the system and all of its components. For example, in front-line practice, piggybacking on what Bill has said, when health care professionals take this family information into account, it changes the type of information they get and they record, whom they talk with in the family, whom they share information with, their assessment of the nature of the problem, the diagnosis, if you will, the type of treatment or care they recommend and whom they involve in that, and the professionals they collaborate with or refer the family to. Those are the implications for front-line practice.

Now, excellent models for family centered practice exist all over. For example, I need to mention that there is a growing new sub-specialty of my own profession of family therapy called medical family therapy. Panelists Bill Doherty and Tom Campbell are leaders in it. Medical family therapists work in collaborative teams with physicians, nurses and others to help treat some of the family behavior patterns and tensions that affect the illness or the course of treatment, to help the family cope with the adjustments and stress dealing with chronic illness.

If you remember, Al Gore spoke enthusiastically at the Democratic Convention about the family therapy his family received to help his whole family deal with the impact on their family of the accident of his young son, and his lengthy hospitalization.

Now, there are other organizations that are working on refining, developing and promoting more family centered care. The Association for the Care of Children's Health has pioneered in helping pediatric hospitals learn how to involve family members in the care of hospitalized children, and they have developed an excellent set of guidelines for hospitals to use to make their whole institution more family centered. There are excellent, well-developed models for providing family centered health and social services to families with children with special health care needs, and to families who are caring for seriously ill members, psychotic members, and members with

Alzheimer's disease. We know how to do family centered care. But these good but isolated family practice models cannot become standard practice without system wide changes, changes in how health care is financed, organized, staffed and delivered.

For example, the patterns of financing health care can make the family centered approach either possible or virtually impossible. The type of insurance coverage, the benefits covered, who is covered in the family, the nature of the claims process all can support or undermine a family centered approach. Current patterns of financing are heavily biased toward expensive, professional and institutional interventions and procedures, and they don't usually support the time needed to work with the families in the ways that Bill and others have discussed. Nor indeed do they pay for the preventive outreach educational programs that are so badly needed for prevention of some of these illnesses and diseases.

The fact that the American health care system relies so heavily on the use of medical specialists, more than any other country, is another major barrier to more holistic family centered approaches, as is the fact that different members of the family are so often treated by different health care providers, and the fact that health care professionals are given so little training in understanding the importance of family factors, or in learning how to mobilize the family to be an active partner in health care. Those who are convinced, as many of us are, that family centered care is more effective also believe that in many cases, it will help to reduce costs.

Now, I return to one of the major gaps in current health care research that hasn't really been talked very much about here. There are very few studies about the effectiveness, and especially the cost effectiveness, of involving family members in health care in the ways we have been talking about. The few we have are very promising, but evaluations of family centered interventions in both physical and mental health care settings are urgently needed.

Now, we do clearly need to learn more about family factors and basic family processes that influence health. I strongly applaud the plans that we are discussing here, to add some sort of more family related questions to the national health interview survey. In addition, Nick Zill urged appropriately that we should do more analysis of existing data sets, and that is really important.

I also want to put in a plug here for more research on marriage. We are all talking about the importance of marriage in how children and adults have better health related outcomes if they are in marriages, but there is surprisingly little research and very little government funding of studies in terms of what makes marriages work, how can we help promote marital stability. Marriage isn't even an entry in the private foundation index. You cannot find a single foundation that is interested in the issue of marriage, which I think says something about where our priorities are, or where our message is.

However, from the immediate policy perspective, although all these things are needed, I do think the research that should have the highest priority is to test in demonstrations of family centered care to determine whether our hunches about cost savings and effectiveness are correct. Only one such major demonstration has ever been launched to my knowledge, and that is the long term care channeling study, which examined home based, community based services for the very frail elderly. Actually, its results were somewhat disappointing from the perspective of cost savings. However, the patients and families much preferred the community based care, even though it was not proved to be less expensive than institutional care. But in spite of this negative finding, what is interesting is, there has been a great expansion of home-based care, so that says something about the influence of research on policy, perhaps. It is a very small, special population. I don't think the results of this study should stop us from thinking that family centered care would not be cost effective.

Mounting family centered care demonstrations may seem an overwhelmingly complicated task, but I wanted to remind you that the strong political and popular support given to the Head Start program rests on a very slim research foundation, namely in one well designed study of a small sample of under 80 children attending a super deluxe model of preschool intervention that only distantly resembles what we actually call the current Head Start programs. I think the point to learn from that is that when the climate is right and the program seems to make good sense, you don't need a huge body of research to convince policy makers this is the right direction to go. So maybe all we need is one or two such studies, and the policy makers and mainstream health care professionals may stand up and take note.

Now, I don't want to sound naive. The shift we are talking about to family centered care would be profound, and it would take decades to accomplish, even if we were fully committed to it. But at least I think we need to start moving in the right direction.

Now, the second issue that I want to talk about is the issue of how we can coordinate and make better use of the data we already collect. At the Family Impact Seminar we have been concerned with these data issues about families since we started in 1976. I came across in our historical files the other day a memorandum that our prestigious advisory group of seminar members wrote to Vice President Mondale in May of 1978, entitled "Federal Data Regarding Families." He was impressed enough with the memo that we all trooped over to the White House and had a very interesting two-hour meeting with him to discuss our concerns and recommendations.

What was interesting and encouraging to me was that although Mondale did not, as far as I know, take any direct action, some of the problems we identified in this memo are being taken care of or have been taken care of. We now do have the major longitudinal survey we felt was so important in the National Health Interview Survey, and thank heavens, the second wave has been funded. We do have the Survey of Income and Program Participation. We complained in this memo that government surveys seldom separately identified data for Hispanics and other ethnic groups, and this definitely would be an improvement on this issue and now they are so identified. There really has been some progress.

But I think there has been much less progress on one of the major problems we identified in this memo in 1978: the fragmentation of data across so many different federal agencies and offices — and I think maybe it has gotten worse, just because there is so much more research going on in this field of family and child research.

At the time we suggested that a task force be formed to identify and make recommendations on how federal data sources should be coordinated and improved. About ten years later, three years or so ago, several members of the Consortium of Family Organizations started a series of meetings in Washington with federal statistics officials and with others to explore again some of these issues of the fragmentation of federal statistics on families.

Once again, collectively we identified a whole range of problems, gaps and inadequacies, which covered many program areas, but generally applied to the health area as well. We noted that child and family related data are collected by at least eight federal departments. Within each department, several dozen offices and agencies are involved. They have very little communication with each other, and they are often unaware of the research that is being conducted by other offices and other agencies. Most of these data collection efforts are program related and collect data only about individuals. This fragmentation results in many serious problems, gaps, duplications and missed opportunities.

I have here a list of the issues we identified, but most of them have been mentioned one way or another, so I won't go over that now. In the course of these discussions, we were encouraged by Herman Haberman, the director of the office of statistics at OMB, to think about whether the relatively new Inter-Agency Forum on aging-related statistics constituted a model that we could adapt to the family field. He felt that this might be a first step, and might create a structure that could begin to work on these complex issues we have been identifying. After several more discussions and the interest and support of many people like Katherine Wolman, who now has Haberman's job, we concluded that a Federal Inter-Agency Forum on Family Statistics looked as if it might be a good idea. If it were provided with some staff support and a limited budget, it could, we believe, serve a really useful purpose and be a catalyst for progress on many of the issues we've been discussing these last couple of days.

We envisaged that such a family-related forum would consist of representatives of all the key federal family related data offices, particularly including some of the policy research offices, such as ASPE. It would include the heads of key agencies and it would also include OMB in its membership, to ensure there was strong leadership and executive support for any of the recommendations that came out of it.

To ensure that the federal officials were fully informed by the concerns of users, we suggested that the forum include a few representatives of national organizations concerned with this issue of federal family data and research. To ensure that it heard from the concerns of the family research community, it should have sufficient budget to bring them in for occasional meetings, special task forces, or conferences such as these.

Now, what could such a forum do? The forum would meet regularly, and subcommittees would work to conduct special tasks and projects in between meetings. The agenda for such a forum would clearly grow and develop in many different directions. The first task might be to get to know each other, identify, and describe what each office is doing and publish an annotated directory which could be made available to others outside government. Indeed, the Child Trends new guide to family data is a fantastic background document for such a forum, both for the people within the federal government and for those outside, and I think we're all looking forward to it enormously.

The forum could then move on to develop special cooperative projects, developing some consistency of definitions and better measures to be used across all agencies, exploring new methodologies, new items to insert in surveys such as these constructs of family strengths we've been talking about, and piggybacking on each other's surveys. I'm aware that these kinds of collaborations do happen occasionally, but it is not part of an ongoing plan of a group of people meeting together regularly.

In the long run, my vision is that it might lead to the production of something like an annual report on the state of families, much like the Council of Economic Advisors has an annual report on the state of the economy, synthesizing and pulling together what we are learning in the whole range of areas. It could conduct some special cross-cutting studies, and publish synthesis reports summarizing the knowledge on the issues of current concern to the public, for example, the effects of divorce and marital stress on children.

These reports would be primarily geared to the public and policy makers, not to other researchers. I think you are fairly good at communicating with each other, although I know communication is often fragmented by discipline, but it is for all the other people who need your information that I make this plea.

COFO very much wanted to help make such a forum a reality, because everyone seemed to think one way or another it made a lot of good sense. We were unfortunately unable to get the funding to continue to do the kind of work, the advocacy work, that was necessary to make it happen. However, meanwhile, the first step was actually already taken by Patrick Fagin at ASPE, who in October of 1991 put together a family data working group, which has about 60 members from offices across HHS. They have been meeting monthly for over a year. I've attended one of their meetings, and I believe the members of this group have found it to be very valuable. Many are here and they can speak for themselves.

There is a new Administration and a new Congress in town, and we hope they will be receptive to such an idea. Since coordination of family data is hardly a partisan issue, I must say I'm optimistic. In my view, it should be expanded to include representatives of other departments and from outside the government. To achieve its full potential, it will need some financial resources from somebody, the agencies or from the Hill.

Finally, I just want to say that I applaud your linking concerns about family data and health to policy. Too often, the fields of research and policy are worlds apart. I wish there had been more members of the policy community present. I wish that the ASPE people hadn't been too busy on welfare and health care reform to be here, but I think I can count on the process to get the information from the conference into their hands.

REFERENCE

Consortium of Family Organizations. (1992, Winter). Principles of family-centered health care: A health reform white paper. *Family Policy Report,* 2:2.

MARILYN COLEMAN, ED.D.
Professor of Human Development and Family Studies
University of Missouri

Family Research, A Basis for Survey Design

In her book, *The Way We Never Were: American Families and the Nostalgia Trap*, published last fall, Stephanie Coontz says many ideas about American families are informed less by reality than by old television shows such as "Leave It to Beaver" and "The Donna Reed Show." Coontz also determined, from her study of the history of American families from 1600 to 1900, that there is no one family form that has ever protected people from poverty, social disruption, or disease, and no traditional arrangement provides a workable model for how we might organize family relations in the modern world.

As Coontz and others make clear, we must reconsider our definitions of families and what they do. It has been suggested that we should think of the family in the same way that we think of the economy. Thinking about the economy does not bring to mind our favorite clothing store at the mall or Walmart headquarters in Benton, Arkansas. We think, instead, of the complexity of organizations and activities having to do with the production and distribution of goods.

Similarly, we should think of the family as the complexity and organization of activities such as family obligations, marriage, parenthood, child-rearing, sibling relationships, inheritance, and health maintenance. We should think beyond our own family or the idealized families of television to the more complex array of modern American families.

The challenges presented by that complexity, however, become almost overwhelming. The difficulty is in designing studies or surveys that adequately assess or even identify all the possible different relationships that might exist in a family. To begin to face up to this difficulty, it is important that family researchers be involved in the design of major surveys sponsored or conducted by the government. Without the advantage of the many painful lessons family researchers have learned while floundering in data representing "new" or "modern" families, survey data are likely to lack elements needed to fully research empirical questions designed to tap important family issues. The examples I offer are primarily from the perspective of a stepfamily researcher, which I am, and I use these examples because stepfamilies are perhaps the most complex of modern American families.

A skilled statistician I often work with told me that as far as data analysts were concerned, stepfamilies should not be allowed to exist! The "if-then" statements needed for the computer to determine such information as the oldest child still living in the household and whom that child belongs to are beyond the pale. Stepfamily complexity has often outwitted the computer! Stepfamilies have also outwitted the Census Bureau. For the first time in history, the 1990 Census asked questions about stepfamily status. Unfortunately, one simple question will not suffice for stepfamilies. In the Census data, a household shows up as a stepfamily household only if the stepparent filled out the form. If the biological parent filled out the form, the stepfamily status was not revealed.

The first wave of the National Survey of Families and Households (NSFH), perhaps the most sophisticated family survey to date, does not allow researchers to distinguish between half-siblings and stepsiblings in the household. Stepfamily researchers would argue that these two groups are quite different and should be studied separately. Although great care was taken with the NSFH to incorporate stepfamily information (e.g., double sampling of stepfamilies), some important analyses are not possible, perhaps because stepfamily complexity was not completely understood and appropriate allowances were not made for it.

Most social and behavioral scientists acknowledge that the traditional first-married nuclear family is no longer necessarily the norm, but that acknowledgment is often reluctant and accompanied by concern about how other families compare to the traditional family. Far too often when nontraditional family data are collected, it is for the purpose of comparing them to traditional nuclear families to see how they "measure up." My colleague, Larry Ganong, and I have referred to this practice as the deficit-comparison approach (Ganong & Coleman, 1984).

The deficit-comparison approach often blinds people to the complexity of stepfamilies and, as a result, all stepfamily types are grouped together, or structural complexity is reduced through study design or statistical procedures (Coleman & Ganong, 1990). These studies seldom yield fruitful insights because the simplistic designs often employed do not allow researchers to rule out the possibility that results are due to unmeasured variables related to family structural variations or family processes.

In addition to careful attention to family structure variations and differences in family processes, survey planners should consider family theory. David Olson referred to the problem of lack of theory in the published family research in his presentation. In my role as editor of the *Journal of Marriage and the Family*, one of the most common complaints of reviewers is that researchers are not using theory to guide their efforts. If surveys have input from family theorists who, unfortunately, are often not the same group as the family researchers, the data are far more likely to be amenable to theoretically sound research. Demographers also are not necessarily theorists, and although their input is crucial to the design of surveys, the input of family demographers alone may not be enough. Even when theory is considered, it is currently unknown whether theoretical propositions that are applicable to nuclear families are also applicable to stepfamilies, single-parent families, and other families.

Whether dealing with theory or empirical data, it is problematic when working with one population to assume that what is found can be generalized to others. A related concern is the common assumption that measures designed and formed on one kind of family will work equally well with other kinds of families.

As David Olson emphasized in his presentation, surveys need to build in measures that have known psychometric properties and less often rely on single items to represent complex variables. However, it cannot be assumed that even measures with known psychometric properties are appropriate to use with stepfamilies or single-parent families if they were normed on nuclear families.

Bill Doherty stressed the importance of the family-and-health interaction, and, of course, that relationship is also affected by family structure changes. What used to be a simple question — "Who is responsible for the health needs of this child?" — is no longer simple. Responsibility could fall to the biological parents, the non-custodial parent, the stepparent, the grandparents, or any combination of these and others — and the combinations will likely change over time.

There are often more health decision makers in these so-called "new" families and questions such as, "Whose health insurance will pay?" are not easily and simply answered. Parents argue incessantly about these issues, perhaps indicating that health care coverage for nontraditional families should be more flexible. Even questions such as, "How many times has this child been to the doctor in the past year?" may be impossible to determine in nontraditional families. For example, the non-custodial parent may have taken the child to the doctor when the child was visiting and not shared the information with the custodial parent. Traditional questioning techniques are often not effective with nontraditional families.

Philip Cowan (1993) recently made an important case for studying families in a more effective way. He says, "We must begin to account not only for the rules but also for the exceptions to the rules, . . . Why is it that some families are more resilient than their life circumstances would suggest? Why are other families, which appear to be in the category that we would label advantaged, vulnerable to what seems like mild stressors? Attempts to answer these questions force us to pay more attention to the specificity and particularity of family life" (p. 470). David Olson's (1991) MASH model is a valiant attempt to get at those issues, but I'm not sure David would suggest he is yet able to comfortably answer those questions.

We need to know how and why families differ across family structure, geographic region, ethnic and cultural background, and in stages of the life cycle. The purpose of this knowledge is not to determine which family is best at providing for optimal health needs or any other variable that might be studied. The object is to determine how different families provide for the optimal development of their members.

Unfortunately, family researchers tend to focus on the negative effects of family change on development. For example, it is usually the negative effects of divorce that are studied. Does divorce always have a negative effect on the health of a family? Feminist family researchers might suggest that the stress of maintaining a traditional family takes a negative toll on women's health; or that women or men who hold families together against all odds may actually be engaging in pathology.

Family researchers need to be more careful than we have been in the past in making assumptions about families. Our reliance on means and averages provides us with valuable information, but tells us little about the unusually resilient family or the family whose coping skills fall far below average. We need to study the statistical outliers, those families who do not perform as we expect. Instead of eliminating these families from our analyses, we need to study them carefully — we may have much to learn from them.

The availability of data from large surveys far too often fosters mindless number crunching. With no theoretical framework as a guide, the number crunchers over and over and over again compare nuclear families or children in nuclear families to other families or children in other fam-

ilies. What does this tell us? How does this help American families? Surveys need to be planned that can provide guidance — how can the negative consequences of family change be minimized? How can positive consequences of family change be identified and maximized? These issues relate quite directly to health care and well-being.

Finally, the designers of surveys need to be aware of the biases that drive the questions they ask; those who analyze and report the data need to realize the biases that drive their methods as well. If we are to have useful data for understanding families and developing policy, we must have input from family researchers who do not have a limited conceptualization of family structure and family process variables nor a deficit-comparison approach to the study of families. Including scholars who are well-versed in the issues of family complexity is a necessary planning step to providing useful data that can answer crucial questions relating to family health policy.

REFERENCES

Coleman, M., & Ganong, G. (1990). Remarriage and stepfamily research in the 1980s: Increased interest in an old family form. *Journal of Marriage and the Family, 52,* 925-940.

Coontz, S. (1992). *The way we never were.* New York: Basic Books.

Cowan, P., Hansen, D., Swanson, G., Field, D., & Skolnick, A. (1993). Issues in defining a research agenda for the 1990s. In P. Cowan, D. Field, D. Hansen, A. Skolnick, & G. Swanson (Eds.), *Family, self, and society: Toward a new agenda for family research.* Hillsdale, NJ: Lawrence Erlbaum.

Ganong, L., & Coleman, M. (1984). Effects of remarriage on children: A review of the empirical literature. *Family Relations, 33,* 389-406.

Olson, D., & Stewart, K. (1991). Family systems and health behaviors. In H. Schroeder, (Ed.), *New directions in health psychology assessment.* New York: Hemisphere.

ROBERT BLUM, M.D., M.P.H., PH.D.
Professor and Director
Division of General Pediatrics and Adolescent Health
University of Minnesota

Critical Issues for the Family Research Agenda and their Use in Policy Formulation

I am a pediatrician. I come with a public health and particularly maternal and child health orientation. My work is primarily in two areas: adolescent sexuality and chronic illness. It is relevant in the comments that I'll be making to have a sense of the perspective that I bring.

One of the things that I have seen over the past decade is that there has been a rise in the rhetoric of family centered care which, in the work that I do, is simplistically equated to in-home care. I think that what has motivated in-home care over the last decade primarily has been economics. The perceived economics of in-home care has been that it is cheaper to take care of people in homes than outside of homes. It is not politically correct to challenge that underlying assumption. It isn't even politically correct to say that it is the underlying assumption, but I think it is.

So when we talk about "family centered care" over the next decade, part of the question for me is, what are we talking about? As I said, I come with a maternal and child health orientation, because I think that in some sectors, when family centered care is discussed, it isn't family centered care; it is maternal centered care, and the male is pretty irrelevant. I'll talk a bit more about that in a minute.

I think we need to look at what the costs are of family centered care, and who bears the costs. What are the opportunity costs? What are the time costs? What are the emotional costs, especially in dealing with family members, and particularly children and youth who have disabling conditions and chronic illnesses? Are these costs equally spread across the family or are they disproportionately clustered? Who are the beneficiaries of family centered care? How are the benefits measured? What do we know about the costs to those who deliver the care? What do we know about the costs to family members who deliver the care, and how does that influence the cost of care in the public and private sectors? Does it reduce it? Does it increase it? While it may decrease the cost of care of the identified individual with the chronic illness or disability, it may also increase the cost of care to other family members less visible, unless the entire family is the unit of analysis.

Within this construct there are also some ethical questions: Who should be the primary beneficiary of family centered care, when there is not a harmony of interest among all members of the family? The notion of "family centered" assumes a harmony of interest, but should the primary beneficiary be the involved member? The child, for example, with the disability? Or is it his or her parents? or the siblings? I think that if we are going to move this notion a step further, we also need to look at some of those very complex ethical issues.

We need to look at these issues in a broader context as well, and that is the context of informal support networks within the community and within religious organizations. To accomplish this, there is a need to develop new models of analysis. For example, some of the work that Linda Burton at Penn State is doing is beginning to move in the direction of new ways of exploring informal support networks.

Another critical question is: What are the service delivery options available to the involved member of a family, when in-home care does not equal family centered care? These are issues that are just beginning to be thought about.

Another set of issues that was raised for me in listening to the discussions this afternoon has to do with the language of "culturally sensitive" delivery of health services, or, what some call "cultural competence." We know that the family is the mediator of culture, and we intuitively know that culture has a dramatic impact on one's understanding of him or herself as a healthy or sick individual. Yet we know little or nothing about the interrelationships between culture, chronic illness, families, and the outcomes for people with disabilities who are covered within one or more cultures concurrently. What are the methodologies that will move us further in those directions? I think these are issues that clearly need to be on the research docket.

A third set of issues was triggered by comments that both David Olson and Bill Doherty made having to do with adolescent risk behaviors, specifically, conflict and cigarette smoking and the inter-correlations between cigarette smoking in parents and children. We just finished an analysis of children who had intercourse below the age of ten. Based on our Minnesota survey of 36,000 kids, we found that about four percent of youths reported having had intercourse below the age of ten. We separated everyone who had indicated they had been sexually abused, about a third of the sample, and analyzed about a thousand young people who said they had had intercourse below the age of ten and had not been sexually abused. We wanted to know, who are these kids? We found that these young people are very different from kids who have intercourse at the age of 12. There is far more family pathology, more family drinking, parental drinking, and parental marijuana use. These kids are far less likely to have an identified adult with whom they relate. They are four times more likely to be failing in school and 15 times more likely to wind up being

pregnant than those who had intercourse at the age of 12 or later.

So what we are seeing is that some of the very basic assumptions, at least some of our basic assumptions about adolescent behaviors, pertain to teenagers at much lower ages than previously considered. When I think about the things that to me needs to be on the agenda, one of the things that to me needs to be considered is understanding adolescent risk behaviors at ages much younger than adolescence, eight to 12 years of age, of which we know very little. There is growing evidence that large numbers of youths are participating in risk behaviors during childhood.

We need to better understand why some kids raised in disadvantaged environments —disadvantaged because of parental alcohol use, disadvantaged because of poverty, because of their own physical impairments, et cetera — go on and do well. I think Dr. Coleman spoke on some of the issues related to resilience. Why do young people who grow up in families where both parents smoke, not grow up to be smokers? Why do some young people who grow up in abusive families not become abusers? The whole area of protective factors is one that is beginning to be explored, but I think therein lie some of the keys to interventions.

We need to better understand how families change over time. It is in how conflict is negotiated, how change is negotiated over time within families that lies our key to understanding of resilience. How are crises dealt with? Crises of the diagnosis of illness? The loss of a job? Puberty? A child's leaving home? We need to more closely examine the major change periods in the lives of families, in particular families with special situations or special needs.

Finally, returning to something I mentioned earlier over the past day and a half: the issue of the marginalization of the male has repeatedly arisen; this is reaffirmed by this view. Research on teen fathers has shown us pretty clearly that about half of all teen fathers stay involved some way or another with their partners. My colleague, Lynn Beringer, and I just finished a study looking at an eight-year follow-up of teenagers who had abortions. These young women are now in their early to mid-twenties. Nearly half of them are still involved with their partners by whom they became pregnant eight years ago. Some of them are married, some were married and are now divorced; some of them maintain friendships. These findings are extraordinary, for the "absent mate" is a myth; yet I couldn't imagine that there are five abortion clinics in the United States that create a welcoming environment for male partners. The same can be said of pregnancy clinics and adoption centers, et cetera. We need a much broader definition, an understanding of the adolescent male, and to develop strategies for his inclusion in services. We need to better understand male sexual behavior data that currently suggest that the mean age of intercourse for the adolescent males is 13.4 years. Is it that they are lying? Is it true? Is it fantasy? What is going on with these data, and how does it differ among various communities and various cultures? When we talk about interventions without knowing what that means, how can we be at all successful?

The issues are clearly very complex, but I think, as Theodora Ooms suggested, that in the final analysis, if we are going to be successful in converting research to the benefit of people and to the benefit of kids, we need to translate that complexity to make it simple, so policy makers can hear it.

IRA KAUFMAN, M.D.
Clinical Associate Professor
University of Medicine & Dentistry of New Jersey

Co-Director
Information for State Health Policy Programs
Robert Wood Johnson Medical School

Family Research in State and Local Policy Making

I am one of the unusual people attending the meeting, because my work is not directly related to family issues. What I do and have been doing for a living for the last 20 or so years has been trying to help state government turn data into information for policy. From that, I have developed a unique perspective on this type of problem.

First of all, you need to understand how policy is made at the state level. More and more, health policy is being generated at the state level instead of the federal level. The way you communicate research findings to these individuals is different; their needs are different. The first rule within government is, all politics are local. If you cannot speak to them in terms of their problems for their specific communities, in terms of what the level in the community is and how that level deviates from what is expected, you cannot get their attention. They need to know how the specific problems that you are concerned about in terms of your family research relates to their community. They have more needs facing them than the funds available. They know what is going on *right now*. It is simply small area analysis at a community level; their community, not your definition of their community.

The second thing that they want from us on a regular basis is timely information, so they have it when they are making their decisions. They do not have large staffs to review literature, to syn-

thesize research and put it together for them. They need it broken down in a time frame that meets their needs.

To make this painfully obvious, let me relate a story related to maternal and child health. It will give you an idea of the current perspective that is going on with state government. We had a conversation going about high rates of infant mortality, why this was an important problem, how the trends had changed, and what it meant for racial and ethnic groups. We had a legislator who had some advisors in from business and labor, and they wanted to know what the infant mortality was last week.

Why don't we know it? If we think it is an important piece of information, why aren't we timely? Why are we talking about something five years ago? Why are we talking about something ten years ago when we are developing a new policy? If we want to be able to track these issues, systems that are responsive in a timely manner to decision makers who commit resources are becoming more and more necessary, which means some integration of the way we go about collecting and analyzing information. Clearly, we have to have it in the can before they ask for it. We need to anticipate it. Mechanisms to bring consensus about what is collected are going to become necessary. These things will need to be put together at national, regional and state levels.

113

Notice I didn't mention the word accuracy of the information. They are not concerned with the accuracy of the information. If we can detect a two percent difference between risk populations, their reaction from the policy maker's perspective is, so what? They're not sure if it's measurement error. In any case, it is not a large percentage of their constituency. They're not going to focus on it. However, there is an audience for that small difference, and that is our program people at state and federal levels who are responsible for designing programs to implement the policies the legislatures believe are important. What they focused on is the targeting of resources to the high risk populations. A two percent difference or a five percent difference in risk populations is relevant information for them.

Frequently we package our information at a very detailed level for policy audiences. The message here is, you've got to package information differently, depending upon your audience. Understand your audience, understand how they look at things. Legislators do not use the mind-set in which I was trained. They certainly do not analyze the situation, look at potential interventions, design strategies and evaluate how successful they are.

They identify a problem, look to see if there is a consensus, act and move on to the next problem. If they didn't do it right, they get another shot at it if they're re-elected. But the sure way they won't be re-elected is not reacting when a problem is identified. Why do we approach them from an analytic perspective in terms of the information provided to them? You are not likely to get the resources in your state to modify programs that you're probably interested in. We all work with community programs as well as our general research area. It is necessary at a state level to secure the funds that flow within your state, since most health policies being generated today are at the state level, and if my reading of the current Administration is correct, it is not likely to move too far from a state level implementation of policy. I think it is necessary that a consensus is put together.

We have heard talk in the previous session about the need for more complex indicators, indices instead of a single measure. I submit to you, when you go to your legislature, you're going to lose them if you use that approach. But the point I tried to make earlier was, accuracy is not the necessary issue here. We do not have to precisely measure the prevalence in the community in their area. We need to monitor how it is changed. It can be a bias indicator.

To put your research into program, however, more detailed information is necessary. You may need your indices at that level. Reliability becomes much more important when we go to implement programs, and knowing how things are actually put together. But the legislature can be handed some very simple numbers that are collected at geographic areas of relevance: congressional districts, assembly districts, and census track level. Ecological relationships work with the legislature for getting them to commit resources, to understand that this is a large problem in their area, or it is not a large problem.

I submit to you that you have to tell them where they are and how they compare with the normative group. For policy at a state level, that normative group may not be the state average, mind you. It may be the federal region, the surrounding states, the nation as a whole. If you try to put together a policy based on how things deviate from the norm within your state, you automatically have half your legislators liking where they stand and half of them not liking where they stand. The benchmark becomes important! Is it the appropriate meter to create the demand for new or reallocated resources?

One of the places I think this group can be very useful in helping to get things going in terms of family level analysis is by putting together some standardized roster of how to go about collecting the demographic and relational information that is necessary for describing families, at the minimal level. Some of you may want to do more detailed breakouts of sub-categories, but if our research starts coming together with larger aggregates that states can monitor, you have some basis for educating your legislature about family issues.

Let us turn to the national health interview survey for a second. One of the primary ways states collect information about their general population is by health interview surveys, sometimes through the National Center for Health Statistics, sometimes independently. There is no standard demographic base module that is collected among the states, because there has been no clear federal leadership as to what that base module should contain. There is probably a willingness for many of the states to pick up that type of information as a model. I submit to you, it is something to provide them to make it easier for them, versus requiring it.

I believe that health interview surveys, behavioral risk factor surveys, and adolescent health surveys are an effective way for monitoring issues at the regional or state levels, and potentially at the sub-state level. But I think most importantly, consensus must be reached in the field as to what that categorization system is, because without it, we're going to get contradictory requests to state government and to the federal government in terms of the classification. As long as that occurs, no funds will come forward for the research, because nobody will quite know what they are going after.

It is much easier for the Congress and Senate to sit back and say when you have a consensus, we'll want to address that issue. But until such time, they will sit back. Consensus is very important in terms of policy at the state level around family issues, around chronic disease. They act based on consensus because there is no risk from a political perspective.

You need to come together as a group and put together a classification system which can be further sub-divided for individual pieces of research, but with a minimum set of relationships that are collected surveys.

Finally, to the extent that your individual research agendas within your institutions can build a roster of information in terms of family relations, states can take that information using indirect standardization techniques to make estimates of detailed information. But by and large, the policy issue comes from our aggregate dependent measures. They are not going to be interested in terms of the fine detail at policy levels. I think a more integrated approach for collecting the information from the local community through the federal level is necessary to create interest in terms of family policy.

MARY GRACE KOVAC, PH.D.
Special Assistant for Data Policy and Analysis
National Center for Health Statistics

Summary

I would like to expound briefly on the meaning of "timeliness" in data dissemination. Please remember that "timely" to policymakers means getting the information when they need it, whereas researchers perceive timeliness as getting data processed and out rapidly.

The issue of national sampling frames being used for state projections was raised by Dr. Peter Benson. Dr. Ira Kaufman explained that federal surveys are designed to efficiently answer federal questions and health policy tends to be at the regional and state levels. For the most part, national surveys cannot be used for making state estimates.

There is a need for different surveys to be unified in some format so that common data may be scrutinized, keeping in mind that generalizations cannot not be made when different sample designs have been used. In fact, there are state level data sets that could be brought together and yield a great deal of information. As Dr. Ooms pointed out, state legislation often represents the crux of family policy.

Dr. Kaufman used the Behavioral Risk Factors Survey and the Adolescent Health Survey as examples of bringing states together to identify survey questions. While this coordinates information across states, the change of questions through the years results in lack of trend data.

Smaller states do not have the resources to conduct large complex surveys. They could benefit from funding and/or coordinated efforts with federal agencies. Dr. Marc Berk from Project Hope noted that due to sampling issues, elaborate surveys for small states would be very difficult. For this reason, he suggests benefits would be realized if federal surveys could somehow flag certain variables, without confidentiality violations, to allow analysis of policy issues. For example, flag those who live in a state with a liberal Medicaid program to better analyze their ecological environment.

Dr. Kaufman emphasized the expense involved in conducting a survey like the National Health Interview Survey due to its size and the fact that it is household based. To be realistic from a state perspective, he questions if a smaller version could be used as a telephone survey, funded by individual states. But, there is an issue of whether state funds can be used for this type of effort. Perhaps federal and state agencies could work together on this so that both would obtain survey data applicable to their policy decision processes.

Members of the panel felt the need to make a distinction between the two terms "family friendly" and "family centered" care. Family centered care must be thought out philosophically regarding its implementation. It must not be like the deinstitutionalization of the mentally ill, where families had no training in support mechanisms and thus, many released patients became homeless. In other words, we should not move too quickly from data to policy without first considering the theoretical and ethical underpinnings.

116

PETER BENSON, PH.D.
President
Search Institute, Minneapolis, MN

Conclusions and Recommendations

BACKGROUND

Co-Sponsors

The Workshop on Family Data and Family Health Policy was co-sponsored by the National Center for Health Statistics, Centers for Disease Control and Prevention; Office of the Assistant Secretary for Health and Human Services; and the Office of the Assistant Secretary for Planning and Evaluation, Department of Health and Human Services.

Participants

The participating scholars and researchers were as follows:

Gerry Hendershot, Presiding
Edward Anthony
Manning Feinleib
Karl Zinsmeister
Edward Schor
Frances Goldscheider
James House
Brent Miller
Nicholas Zill
John S. Lyons
Ron Haskins
Kristin Moore
Jack Feldman
David Olson
William Doherty
Theodora Ooms
Marilyn Coleman

Robert Blum
Ira Kaufman
Peter Benson
Thomas Campbell
Elizabeth Thomson
David Williams

Workshop Purposes

The workshop was guided by three overall purposes:

- To identify important emerging family-related public health issues
- To identify the health data most needed for policy on those issues
- To recommend practical steps needed to produce those health data

Conclusions and Recommendations

This report summarizes workshop conclusions and recommendations per the third purpose listed above.

Following two days of presentations and focused discussions, conference participants were asked to write a response to this question: "What conclusions and recommendations should emerge from this conference?" These responses were then synthesized and presented to workshop participants for discussion, elaboration, and refinement, with the intent of generating consensus. The following pages capture the essence of this consensus-building process. It is divided into four parts:

117

Facilitator

The four participants who facilitated this process were:

Peter Benson, Search Institute (Chair)
Thomas Campbell, University of Rochester School of Medicine
Elizabeth Thomson, University of Wisconsin
David Williams, University of Michigan

PART I: CONFERENCE CONCLUSIONS

In discussing family data and health policy, several key assumptions guided participants' collective thinking:

- Families have a profound influence on health. This relationship has not been fully explored.
- Both health policy and its effectiveness can be dramatically informed by family data. Currently, however, limitations in the scope and quality of federal family data systems undermine this potential.
- The connection of family data to health policy could be maximized if each of the 18 conclusions listed below are heeded. Each of these is attainable, but will require the development of new procedures, stronger linkages to university researchers, and improved coordination that can ultimately be cost-effective.

Definitions

1. Think expansively. Traditional definitions of family, which often center on adult care-givers living with children, are constricting. It is more useful to view all citizens as family members. Even those who live alone need to be seen as part of a family, since relationships with family members, whether proximate or distal, inform health status and health outcomes.
2. Develop new family definitions. New conceptual work on the formal definition of family is needed. Definitions based on blood, marriage, or adoption do not provide inclusivity or flexibility needed to capture the wide range of care-giving arrangements now evidenced in U.S. society.
3. Carefully define the territory of "health" issues.

Measurement

4. Measure structure and process. Federal research pays more attention to family structure than to family process or dynamics. Family issues such as support, conflict, cohesion, communication, flexibility, and satisfaction.
5. Develop more psychometrically-sound measurement tools.
6. Develop more concise measurement of key constructs, without sacrificing psychometric soundness.
7. Develop more theory-driven and policy-driven measurement tools.

Design

8. Collect data on multiple family members.
9. Design surveys so that family members can be linked, permitting family to serve as the unit of analysis.

Context

10. Assess the contextual factors (economics, community, neighborhood) which shape family structure and process.
11. Assess life cycle differences in health status, health outcomes, and family impact.

Diversity

12. Pay more rigorous attention to cultural diversity in family structure *and* process.

Sampling and Data Collection

13. Pay more attention to including males in national data collections.
14. Develop sampling frames which permit reliable state estimates.

Family Cohesion

15. Monitor the factors known to promote

marital and family stability. Such stability has a major impact on health.

Health-Care Delivery

16. Monitor the interactions of families and family members with health care professionals.
17. Evaluate the role of family-centered health delivery models.

Coordination

18. Increase federal coordination of family data systems and policy formation.

PART II: RECOMMENDATIONS ON WHAT HEALTH ISSUES SHOULD BE INFORMED BY FAMILY DATA

Health Promotion

1. Shift some energy to positive health behaviors (e.g., nutrition, fitness).
2. Expand to include mental health issues.

Prevention

3. Monitor family experiences with violence, both inside and outside the family context.
4. Emphasize illnesses known to be preventable.
5. Monitor early onset of risk behaviors, in the 8-12 age range.
6. Monitor adolescent driving behaviors (e.g., accidents, driving and drinking).
7. Study the interconnection of adolescent risk behaviors.

Access

8. Monitor family contact with "family-friendly" health delivery.
9. Monitor family members' access to insurance benefits.
10. Study family beliefs about health care and their perceived accessibility and efficacy; study demand for "nontraditional" care.

Caregiving

11. Monitor chronic conditions requiring constant care.

12. Monitor experiences with disability and rehabilitation.

Family Life

13. Document how families resolve conflict.
14. Document the frequency and health impact of life transitions.
15. Study the impact of illness on other family members.
16. Study the impact of alcohol and other drug use on family members.
17. Study the health consequences of family formation variables (e.g., number of births, spacing, planning, adolescent pregnancy).

Focus

18. In data collection and policy, balance current emphasis on children with emphasis on adults.

Priorities

19. Decisions about what health issues to address should be driven by four criteria:
   • focus on the most vulnerable individuals
   • focus on the most preventable behaviors
   • focus on persons with multiple health problems
   • focus on the health behaviors which, in the aggregate, are most costly to society

PART III: RECOMMENDATIONS ON ENHANCING DATA QUALITY

Improving Survey Content (recommended constructs to be developed and measured)

1. Individuals' perceptions of "who is in my family" (this is viewed as a counterweight to the more traditional measurement of household composition).
2. Family gender roles.
3. Family process (e.g., satisfaction, cohesion, conflict, flexibility, communication, marital satisfaction).
4. Family beliefs, attitudes, and values about health.
5. Role of stepparents.
6. Role of biological parents who do not reside with birth children.
7. Family transition and history.
8. Experience with family-centered providers.

9. Economic and cultural variations in structure and process.
10. Intergenerational connections (e.g., communication, caregiving, income transfer).
11. Indicators of marital stability.
12. Parental conflict, family violence, and family procedures for conflict resolution.
13. Insurance coverage.
14. Caregiving: forms of receiving, forms of giving.

Measurement/Psychometrics

1. Investigate psychometric properties of current measures.
2. Develop concise and psychometrically sound measures of key constructs; validate across multiple racial-ethnic categories (extensive research needed *before* inclusion in federal surveys).
3. Tie measurement to theory and literature.
4. Validate self-reports of service receipt.
5. Disseminate research findings; make easily available to researchers and general public.
6. Build research capacity on "staff."
7. Conduct research on how to create multiple data linkages within families.

Data Management/Data Collection

1. Standardize family indicators across federal data collections.
2. Survey multiple family members, link data while preserving confidentiality.
3. Identify family types not currently captured and develop appropriate strategies.
4. Develop strategies to maximize participation of males.
5. Link across data sources.
6. Increase researchers' accessibility to data sets.
7. Make linking of family data more user-friendly.
8. Explore how/whether to link individuals across multiple households.
9. Design population studies to model branching processes.
10. Develop procedures to impute missing family data.

PART IV: RECOMMENDATIONS ON ACTIONS NEEDED TO MAXIMIZE DATA-POLICY CONNECTIONS

Recommendations to Federal Statistical Agencies

1. Intentionally involve more researchers in survey development.
2. Sponsor forums on definitions of family.
3. Sponsor forums on how data can be connected to health policy.
4. Develop mechanisms of communication linking researchers with policymakers at federal and state levels.
5. Develop sampling frames to permit state estimates and/or advocate for state minimal data sets.
6. Quicken reporting.
7. Develop short, user-friendly issue briefs.
8. Sponsor forums on defining family process issues, to be added to federal data collections.

Additional Recommendations to NCHS

9. Include some family variables in the NHIS core model.
10. Support the family health topical module.

Recommendations to Funding Agencies

1. Support innovative research programs to identify health promoting family processes, beliefs, attitudes, values and social contexts.
2. Support consensus-building among researchers on constructs and measurements.
3. Support replication studies.
4. Provide incentives to researchers to validate items and develop concise measures for use in federal surveys.
5. Fund demonstrations and evaluations of family-centered health delivery models.
6. Fund research on the costs of various policy proposals and initiatives.
7. Support dissemination of family research; consider coordination with association journals.

Recommendations, Mechanisms of Coordination

1. Establish a permanent interagency family health data forum (build on ASPE Family

Data Work Group). Include federal agencies, researchers, and associations.

2. Expect this forum to identify a common core of family items for all national surveys, with a process for periodically changing the common core.

3. Promote a national bulletin board.
4. Consider re-establishing a column in *The Journal of Marriage and Family*.
5. Sponsor pre-conference workshops.
6. Ensure inclusion of family items in education and department of justice surveys.

Participant List

Pre-Registered Participants

Edward Anthony, Ph.D.
Director, Policy and Planning
Office of Special Education and Rehabilitative
Services
Department of Education
Humphrey Building, Room 424E
400 Maryland Avenue, S.W.
Washington, DC 20201

Linda Baber
Research Assistant
Robert Wood Johnson Foundation
P.O. Box 2316
Princeton, NJ 08543

Christine Bachrach, Ph.D.
Chief, Demographic and Behavioral Sciences
  Branch
National Institute for Child Health and Human
  Development
Room 8B13
6100 Executive Boulevard
Rockville, MD 20852

Peter Benson, Ph.D.
President
Search Institute
700 South Third Street, Suite 210
Minneapolis, MN 55415

Marc Berk, Ph.D.
Director
Project HOPE: Center for Health Affairs
2 Wisconsin Circle
Chevy Chase, MD 20815

Donald Bloch, M.D.
Director Emeritus
Ackerman Institute for Family Therapy
Editor
Family Systems Medicine
40 West 12th Street
New York, NY 10011

Robert Blum, M.D., M.P.H., Ph.D.
Professor and Director
Division of Pediatric and Adolescent Health
University of Minnesota
Box 721
420 Delaware Street, S.E.
Minneapolis, MN 55455

Barbara Butler
Program Analyst
National Center for Health Statistics
Presidential Building, Room 1100
6525 Belcrest Road
Hyattsville, MD 20782

Thomas Campbell, M.D.
Associate Professor of Family Medicine and
  Psychiatry
University of Rochester
885 South Avenue
Rochester, NY 14620

Marilyn Coleman, Ed.D.
Professor and Chairperson
Human Development and Family Studies
University of Missouri-Columbia
61 Stanley Hall
Columbia, MO 65211

Mary Jo Czaplewski, Ph.D., C.F.L.E.
Executive Director
National Council on Family Relations
Suite 550
3989 Central Avenue, N.E.
Minneapolis, MN 55421

William J. Doherty, Ph.D.
Professor
Family Social Science Department
University of Minnesota
290 McNeal Hall
St. Paul, MN 55108

Jeff Evans, Ph.D., J.D.
Health Scientist Administrator
National Institute for Child Health and Human
   Development
Room 8B13
6100 Executive Boulevard
Rockville, MD 20892

Manning Feinleib, M.D., Ph.D.
Director
National Center for Health Statistics
Presidential Building, Room 1140
6525 Belcrest Road
Hyattsville, MD 20782

Jack Feldman, Ph.D.
Associate Director for Analysis and
   Epidemiology
National Center For Health Statistics
Presidential Building, Room 1000
6525 Belcrest Road
Hyattsville, MD 20782

Margaret Feldman, Ph.D.
Washington Representative
National Council on Family Relations
1311 Delaware Avenue, S.W.
Washington, DC 20024

Frances Goldsheider, Ph.D.
Professor
Brown University/Rand Corporation
1700 Main Street
Santa Monica, CA 90407

Jeanne Griffith, Ph.D.
Associate Commissioner for Data Development
National Center Education Statistics
Room 400
550 New Jersey Avenue, N.W.
Washington, DC 20208-5650

Nancy Hamilton
Public Health Advisor
National Center for Health Statistics
Presidential Building, Room 1100
6525 Belcrest Road
Hyattsville, MD 20782

Ron Haskins, Ph.D.
Welfare Counsel
Committee on Ways and Means
U.S. House of Representatives
1106 Longworth, HOB
Washington, DC 20515

Gerry E. Hendershot, Ph.D.
Chief, Illness and Disability Statistics Branch
National Center for Health Statistics
Presidential Building, Room 850
6525 Belcrest Road
Hyattsville, MD 20782

James S. House, Ph.D.
Professor of Sociology
Director, Survey Research Center
University of Michigan
Institute for Social Research
426 Thompson, Room 3010
P.O. Box 1248
Ann Arbor, MI 48106

Ira Kaufman, M.D.
Clinical Associate Professor
University of Medicine and Dentistry of
   New Jersey
Co-Director, Information for State Health
   Policy Programs
Robert Wood Johnson Medical School
675 Hose Lane
Piscataway, NJ 08854

Mary Grace Kovar, Ph.D.
Special Assistant for Data Policy and Analysis
National Center for Health Statistics
Presidential Building, Room 1120
6525 Belcrest Road
Hyattsville, MD 20782

David Larson, M.D., M.S.P.H.
Senior Policy Analyst
ASPE, DHHS
Office of the Director
National Institutes of Health
Building 31, Room B1-C35
Bethesda, MD 20892

Felicia B. LeClere, Ph.D.
Health Statistician
National Center for Health Statistics
Presidential Building, Room 850
6525 Belcrest Road
Hyattsville, MD 20782

John S. Lyons, Ph.D.
Associate Professor of Psychiatry
Department of Psychiatry
Northwestern University Medical School
303 East Superior Avenue
PAS 584
Chicago, IL 60611

Jennifer Madans, Ph.D.
Acting Director, Division of Analysis
National Center for Health Statistics
Presidential Building, Room 1080
6525 Belcrest Road
Hyattsville, MD 20782

Jane Mauldon, Ph.D., M.P.A.
Assistant Professor/Regional Planning
Graduate School of Public Policy
University of California - Berkeley
2607 Hearst Avenue
Berkeley, CA 94709

Brent C. Miller, Ph.D.
Professor
Department of Family and Human Development
Utah State University
Logan, UT 84322-2905

Kristin Moore, Ph.D.
Executive Director
Child Trends, Inc.
4301 Connecticut Avenue, N.W., Suite 100
Washington, DC 20008

David H. Olson, Ph.D.
Professor
Department of Family Social Science
University of Minnesota
290 McNeal Hall
1985 Buford Avenue
St. Paul, MN 55108

Theodora Ooms, M.S.W.
Director
Family Impact Seminar
American Association for Marriage and Family
Therapy Research and Education Foundation
1100 17th Street, N.W., Suite 901
Washington, DC 20036

William Pratt, Ph.D.
Special Assistant for Family Statistics
National Center for Health Statistics
Presidential Building, Room 830
6525 Belcrest Road
Hyattsville, MD 20782

Martha Riche, Ph.D.
Director, Policy Studies
Population Reference Bureau
Suite 520
1875 Connecticut Avenue, N.W.
Washington, DC 20009

Edward L. Schor, M.D.
Associate Professor of Pediatrics and Community
Medicine
Tufts University Medical School
The Health Institute
New England Medical Center
750 Washington Street
Box #345
Boston, MA 02111

Edward Spar
Executive Director
COPAFS
1429 Duke Street
Alexandria, VA 22314

Elizabeth Thomson, Ph.D.
Professor
Department of Sociology
University of Wisconsin
1180 Observatory Drive
Madison, WI 53706

Debra Umberson, Ph.D.
Associate Professor
Department of Sociology
University of Texas
Burdine Hall, Floor 336
Austin, TX 78712

David R. Williams, Ph.D., M.P.H.
Associate Research Scientist
Associate Professor of Sociology
Institute for Social Research
University of Michigan
P.O. Box 1248
Ann Arbor, MI 48106

Christine Winquist Nord, Ph.D.
Senior Research Scientist
Westat, Inc.
1650 Research Boulevard
Rockville, MD 20850-3129

Nicholas Zill, Ph.D.
Vice President
Westat Inc.
1650 Research Boulevard
Rockville, MD 20850

Karl Zinsmeister, Ph.D.
Adjunct Scholar
American Enterprise Institute
430 South Geneva Street
Ithaca, NY 14850

On-Site Registered Participants

Kay Anderson, M.A.
Statistician
National Center for Health Statistics
Presidential Building, Room 850
6525 Belcrest Road
Hyattsville, MD 20879

Peggy Barker, M.P.H.
Survey Statistician
National Center for Health Statistics/DHIS/SPDR
Presidential Building
6525 Belcrest Road
Hyattsville, MD 20782

Bobbie Bloom, M.P.A.
Statistician
National Center for Health Statistics
Presidential Building
6525 Belcrest Road
Hyattsville, MD 20879

Brett Brown, Ph.D.
Research Associate
Child Trends, Inc.
Suite 610
2100 M Street, N.W.
Washington, DC 20037

Mary Jo Coiro, M.A.
Research Analyst
Child Trends, Inc.
Suite 610
2100 M Street, N.W.
Washington, DC 20037

Ronald Czaja, Ph.D.
Associate Professor
North Carolina State University
Department of Sociology
Box 8107
Raleigh, NC 27695

Margaret Daly
Westat, Inc.
1650 Research Boulevard
Rockville, MD 20850

Heather Ann Davis, Ph.D.
Social Science Research Analyst
Health Care Financing Administration
6325 Security Boulevard
Baltimore, MD 21207

Marjorie Greenberg, M.A.
Evaluation Officer
National Center for Health Statistics
Presidential Building
6525 Belcrest Road
Hyattsville, MD 20879

Ted Greenstein, Ph.D.
Assistant Professor
North Carolina State University
Box 8107
Raleigh, NC 27695

Wilbur Hadden
Statistician
National Center for Health Statistics
Presidential Building
6525 Belcrest Road
Hyattsville, MD 20782

Susan Jack, M.S.
Statistician
National Center for Health Statistics
Presidential Building
6525 Belcrest Road
Hyattsville, MD 20879

Samuel Kessel, M.D., M.P.H.
Director, Div. Systems, Education & Science
MCHB/HRSA/PHS
Parklawn Building, Room 18A55
5600 Fishers Lane
Rockville, MD 20857

John Kiely, Ph.D.
Visiting Scientist
Division of Analysis
National Center for Health Statistics
Presidential Building
6525 Belcrest Road
Hyattsville, MD 20782

5833 009

Kristen Larson, Ph.D.
Social Science Analyst
Division of Family and Community Policy/ASPE
Room 424E
200 Independence Avenue, S.W.
Washington, DC 20201

Donna Ruane Morrison, Ph.D.
Research Associate
Child Trends, Inc.
2100 M Street, N.W.
Washington, DC 20037

Steve W. Rawlings, Ph.D.
Family Demographer
U.S. Census Bureau
Washington, DC 20233-0034

Deborah Rose, Ph.D.
Epidemiologist
National Center for Health Statistics
Presidential Building
6525 Belcrest Road
Hyattsville, MD 20782

Gloria Simpson, M.A.
Statistician
National Center for Health Statistics
Presidential Building
6525 Belcrest Road
Hyattsville, MD 20879

Karen Smith Thiel, Ph.D.
Director, Healthy Start Evaluation
Office of Planning, Evaluation & Legislation
HRSA
Parklawn Building, Room 14-36
Rockville, MD 20857

Barbara Foley Wilson, M.A.
Demographer
National Center for Health Statistics
Presidential Building
6525 Belcrest Road
Hyattsville, MD 20782

DEC 1 6 1994